Basic Allied Health Statistics and Analysis

Gerda Koch

Delmar Publishers

An International Thomson Publishing Company

Albany • Bonn • Cincinnati • Detroit • London • Madrid • Melbourne
Mexico City • New York • Pacific Grove • Paris • San Francisco
Singapore • Tokyo • Toronto • Washington

NOTICE TO THE READER

Publishing Team:
Publisher: David C. Gordon
Acquisitions Editor: Marion Waldman
Editorial Assistant: Sarah Holle
Project Editor: Melissa Conan
Production Coordinator: Mary Ellen Black

COPYRIGHT © 1996
By Delmar Publishers
A division of International Thomson Publishing Inc.

I(T)P The ITP logo is a trademark under license

Printed in the United States of America

For more information, contact:

Delmar Publishers
3 Columbia Circle, Box 15015
Albany, NY 12212-5015

International Thomson Publishing Europe
Berkshire House 168-173
High Holborn
London, WC1V7AA
England

Thomas Nelson Australia
102 Dodds Street
South Melbourne, 3205
Victoria, Australia

Nelson Canada
1120 Birchmount Road
Scarborough, Ontario
Canada M1K 5G4

International Thomson Editores
Compos Eliseos 385, Piso 7
Col Polanco
11560 Mexico D F Mexico

International Thomson Publishing Gmbh
Königswinterer Strasse 418
53227 Bonn
Germany

International Thomson Publishing Asia
221 Henderson Road
#05-10 Henderson Building
Singapore 0315

International Thomson Publishing – Japan
Hirakawacho Kyowa Building, 3F
2-2-1 Hirakawacho
Chiyoda-ku, 102 Tokyo
Japan

1 2 3 4 5 6 7 8 9 10 XXX 02 01 00 99 98 97 96 95

Library of Congress Cataloging-in-Publication Data

Koch, Gerda
    Basic allied health statistics and analysis / by Gerda Koch.
        p.   cm.
    Includes index.
    ISBN 0-8273-5525-4
    1. Medicine—Statistical methods.   2. Public health—Statistical methods.   3. Medical statistics.   I. Title.
    [DNLM: 1. Hospitalization.   2. Statistics—methods.   WX 158 K76d 1996]
R853.S7K63 1996
610'.72—dc20
DNLM/DLC
for Library of Congress   94-23929
                                                                                CIP

Contents

PREFACE   ix

CHAPTER 1   REPORTING STATISTICAL DATA   1

A. **Introduction**...................2
  1. Statistics and Data.............2
  2. Scope of Book.................3
B. **Statistical Data Terms and**
   Definitions...................3
  1. Population vs. Sample...........3
  2. Variable vs. Constant...........4
  3. Qualitative vs. Quantitative
     Variables...................4
  4. Discrete vs. Continuous Data......4
  5. Ungrouped vs. Grouped Data.....4
  6. Descriptive vs. Inferential
     Statistics...................5
C. **Computerized Data**..........5
  1. Use.......................5
  2. Accuracy..................5
D. **Patient Data Collection**..........5

  1. Types of Data Collected..........5
     a. Dates....................6
     b. Counts...................6
     c. Test Results...............6
     d. Diagnosis.................6
     e. Procedures...............6
     f. Treatment Outcomes
        and Assessments............6
E. **Abbreviations**...................7
  1. Patient Care................7
  2. Statistical..................7
  3. Clinical Units...............7
  4. Non-Official Abbreviations........8
F. **Uses of Data**....................8
G. **Summary**......................8
H. **Chapter 1 Test**..................9

CHAPTER 2   MATHEMATICAL REVIEW   11

A. **Fractions**.......................12
  1. Numerator.................12
  2. Denominator................12
  3. Quotient...................13
B. **Decimals**......................13
C. **Percentages**...................13

D. **Rates**.........................13
E. **Ratio**.........................14
F. **Proportion**....................14
G. **Averaging**.....................14
H. **Rounding Data**.................15

I. **Conversion to Another Form**. 17
   1. Fraction to Percentage. 17
   2. Ratio to Percentage. 17
   3. Decimal to Percentage 17
   4. Percentage to Decimal 18
   5. Percentage to Fraction. 18

J. **Computing with a Percentage** 18
K. **Summary** 19
L. **Chapter 2 Test** 20

CHAPTER 3   CENSUS   **22**

A. **Census Collection and Terms**. 23
   1. Census 23
   2. Inpatient Census 23
   3. Hospital Patients 23
      a. Inpatients 23
      b. Outpatients. 23
   4. Hospital Departments 24
   5. Hospital Units vs. Services 24
   6. Clinical Units. 24
   7. Census Taking 24
      a. Time of Day 24
      b. Reporting 25
      c. Central Collection 25
      d. Transfers 25
   8. Admitted and Discharged (A&D). . . 26
   9. Daily Inpatient Census (DIPC) 26
   10. Inpatient Service Day (IPSD) 26
      a. Unit of Measure vs. Totals 27
      b. Period. 27
      c. Synonymous Figures 27
      d. Watch Out 28
   11. Total Inpatient Service Days. 28
      a. Daily Recording—Recording of Daily
          Inpatient Census (DIPC) and
          Inpatient Service Days (IPSD) . . . 28
      b. Example 28
   12. Deaths/Discharges. 28

      a. Included 28
      b. Not Included 29
   13. Census Calculation Tips. 29
   14. Beds/Bassinets. 30
      a. Inpatient Classification
          Categories. 30
      b. Beds 30
      c. Bassinets 30
      d. Adults and Children (A&C) 30
      e. Newborns (NB). 30

B. **Average Census** 32
   1. Average Daily Inpatient Census 32
      a. Explanation. 32
      b. Separate A&C/NB Data. 33
      c. Days in Month 33
      d. Leap Year 33
      e. Rounding 33
      f. Logical Answers. 33
   2. Other Formulae for Census
       Averages 33
      a. A&C 33
      b. NB 34
      c. Clinical Unit 34
   3. Example 34
C. **Summary** 35
D. **Chapter 3 Test** 36

CHAPTER 4   PERCENTAGE OF OCCUPANCY   **40**

A. **Bed/Bassinet Count Terms** 41
   1. Inpatient Bed Count or Bed
       Complement. 41
   2. Newborn Bassinet Count. 41
B. **Rate Formula** 41
C. **Beds** 42
   1. Unit vs. Totals 42
   2. Excluded Beds. 42
   3. Disaster Beds. 42
D. **Bed/Bassinet Count Day Terms**. 42
   1. Inpatient Bed Count Day. 43

   2. Inpatient Bassinet Count Day 43
   3. Inpatient Bed Count Days (Total). . . 43
E. **Occupancy Ratio/Percentage** 43
   1. Adults and Children (A&C) 43
      a. Inpatient Bed Occupancy Ratio . . 43
      b. Formula: Daily Inpatient Bed
          Occupancy Percentage 43
      c. Explanation. 43
      d. All Beds Occupied 43
      e. Disaster Beds and Occupancy
          Rates. 44
      f. Normal Occupancy Percentage. . 44

2. Newborn (NB) 44
   a. Formula: Daily Newborn Bassinet
      Occupancy Percentage 44
   b. Example 44

F. **Occupancy Percentage for a
Period** 45
1. Bed 45

2. Newborn (NB) 46
3. Clinical Unit 46

G. **Change in Bed Count During a
Period** 48
H. **Summary** 50
I. **Chapter 4 Test** 52

CHAPTER 5   MORTALITY (DEATH) RATES   57

A. **Terms** 58
1. Mortality 58
2. Morbidity 58
3. Discharge 58
4. Death 58
   a. Inpatient Death 58
   b. Non-Inpatient Death 59
5. Net vs. Gross 60

B. **Death Rates** 60
1. Gross Death Rate 60
2. Net Death Rate or Institutional
   Death Rate 61
3. Helpful Hints 62

4. Newborn Death Rate 62
5. Surgical Death Rates 65
   a. Postoperative Death Rate 65
   b. Anesthesia Death Rate 66
6. Maternal Death Rate 67
   a. Terms 67
   b. Maternal Deaths Included 68
   c. Deaths Not Included 68
7. Fetal Death Rate 70
   a. Included in Fetal Death Rates . . . 70
   b. Fetal Death Rate Formula 70

C. **Summary** 72
D. **Chapter 5 Test** 73

CHAPTER 6   AUTOPSY RATES   79

A. **Terms/Information** 80
1. Autopsy 80
2. Hospital Autopsy 80
3. Hospital Inpatient Autopsy 80
4. Coroner's/Medical Examiner's
   Cases 80
5. Who Performs an Autopsy 81
6. Hospital Autopsy 81
   a. Who Performs 81
   b. Where 81
   c. Who Is Included 81
   d. Not Included 81
   e. Report Requirements 81

   f. Legal Cases 82
   g. Consent 82
   h. Combine A&C/NB 82

B. **Autopsy Rates** 83
1. Gross Autopsy Rate 83
2. Net Autopsy Rate 85
3. Hospital Autopsy Rate 86
4. Newborn Autopsy Rate 89
5. Fetal Autopsy Rate 90

C. **Summary** 91
D. **Chapter 6 Test** 91

CHAPTER 7   LENGTH OF STAY/DISCHARGE DAYS   95

A. **Terms** 96
1. Length of Stay (LOS)—(For One
   Inpatient) 96
2. Total Length of Stay—(For All
   Inpatients) 96
3. Discharge Days (DD) 96
4. Average Length of Stay 96

B. **Calculating Length of Stay** 96
1. General 96
2. A&D Same Day 97
3. Admitted One Day and
   Discharged the Next 97
4. Longer Stays 97

C. Total Length of Stay 98
   1. Importance of Discharge Days..... 98
   2. Totaling. 98
D. Average Length of Stay 99
   1. Adults and Children (A&C) 100
   2. Newborn (NB) 103

E. Day on Leave of Absence 105
F. Summary 105
G. Chapter 7 Test 106

CHAPTER 8   MISCELLANEOUS RATES   **110**

A. Rates. 111
   1. Cesarean Section Rate. 111
     a. Delivery. 111
     b. Not Delivered 111
     c. Cesarean Section Rate
       Formula 111
   2. Consultation Rate 113
     a. Consultation Rate Formula 114
   3. Infection Rates. 115
     a. Hospital Infection Rate
       Formula 115

     b. Postoperative Infection Rate ... 116
   4. Bed Turnover Rate. 120
     a. Direct Bed Turnover Rate
       Formula 121
     b. Indirect Bed Turnover Rate
       Formula 121
     c. Bassinet Turnover Rate 121
     d. Usefulness of Turnover Rates ... 121
B. Summary 122
C. Chapter 8 Test 123

UNIT I EXAM—CHAPTERS 3 THROUGH 8   **127**

CHAPTER 9   FREQUENCY DISTRIBUTION   **136**

A. Introduction. 137
   1. Ungrouped Frequency
     Distribution. 137
   2. Grouped Frequency
     Distribution. 137
   3. Purpose of a Grouped Frequency
     Distribution 138
     a. Bring Order to Chaos 138
     b. Condense Data to a More Readily
       Grouped Form 138
   4. Arranging Scores. 138
B. Terms Related To a Frequency
  Distribution 138
   1. Range 139
   2. Class 139
     a. Class Interval. 139
     b. Class Limits 140
     c. Class Boundaries 140
     d. Class Size/Class Width....... 140
   3. Frequency. 141
   4. Cumulative Frequency. 141

     a. First Row 141
     b. Second Row 141
     c. Subsequent Rows 141
     d. Top Row 142
C. Creating a Frequency
  Distribution 142
   1. Determine High and Low
     Scores 142
   2. Arrange Scores in Descending or
     Ascending Order. 142
   3. Determine Range 142
   4. Determine the Number of Class
     Intervals 142
   5. Set Class/Score Limits 143
     a. Suggested Methods 143
     b. Departures from Convention... 143
   6. Rules for Subsequent
     Computations 143
D. Summary 146
E. Chapter 9 Test 147

CHAPTER 10   MEASURES OF CENTRAL TENDENCY   **149**

A. **Mean** **150**
  1. Arithmetic Mean 150
  2. Weighted Mean. 150
  3. Mean Computed from Grouped
     Data 151
B. **Median**. **152**
C. **Mode** **152**
D. **Curves of a Frequency Distribution. . 153**
  1. Bilaterally Symmetrical Curves. . . . 153
     a. Bell-shaped Curve 153
     b. Other Symmetrical Curves 153
  2. Skewed Curves 154
     a. Skewed to the Right 154
     b. Skewed to the Left 154
     c. Effect of Skewness on the Measures
        of Central Tendency 155
     d. Reporting Measures of Central
        Tendency from a Skewed
        Distribution. 155
     e. Suggestions for Reporting
        Averages 156
     f. Additional Points. 156
  3. Other Curves. 156
     a. J-Shaped 157

     b. Reversed J-Shaped. 157
     c. U-Shaped 157
     d. Bimodal 157
     e. Multimodal. 157
E. **Ranks/Quartiles/Deciles/Centiles/
   Percentiles** **157**
  1. Terms 158
     a. Rank 158
     b. Quartiles 158
     c. Deciles 158
     d. Centiles/Percentiles 158
     e. Percentile Rank 158
     f. Percentile Score. 158
  2. Percentages/Percentiles. 158
     a. Importance of Percentiles 158
     b. Weakness of Percentiles. 159
     c. Cumulative Frequency Related to
        Percentiles. 159
     d. Conversion of Cumulative
        Frequency into
        Percentage/Percentile 159
F. **Summary** **160**
G. **Chapter 10 Test** **160**

CHAPTER 11   GRAPHING DATA   **163**

A. **Plotting a Frequency Distribution** . . . **164**
  1. Axes 165
  2. Vertical Scale. 165
  3. Scale Proportion 165
B. **Types of Graphs/Charts/Diagrams . . 165**
  1. Histogram. 165
     a. Construction of a Histogram . . . 166
     b. Summary for Constructing a
        Histogram. 167
     c. Variations in Histogram
        Construction. 169
  2. Frequency Polygon 170
     a. Advantage of Frequency
        Polygon 170
     b. When to Use 170
     c. Construction of a Frequency
        Polygon 170

  3. Histogram and Frequency Polygon—
     Additional Information 171
     a. Comparisons. 171
     b. Supplementary Suggestions for
        Construction. 171
     c. Superimposing Figures 171
  4. Bar Graph/Bar Chart 172
     a. Construction of a Bar Graph . . . 173
  5. Line Graph 174
  6. Pie Graph/Pie Chart. 175
  7. Pictograph/Pictogram 177
  8. Comparison Graph: 177
     a. Bar Graphs 178
     b. Line Graphs. 180
C. **Summary** **181**
D. **Chapter 11 Test** **181**

UNIT II EXAM—CHAPTERS 9 THROUGH 11   **186**

APPENDICES

I. DEFINITIONS   **191**

A. Patient Terms 191

B. Inpatient Terms 191

C. Census-Related Terms 192

D. Bed/Bassinet Count Terms 192

E. Occupancy Terms 193

F. Death-Related Terms 193

G. Autopsy Terms 193

H. Length of Stay/Discharge Day Terms 194

I. OB/Maternal Terms 194

J. Newborn Terms 195

K. Miscellaneous Terms 195

II. FORMULAE   **196**

A. Census Formulae 196

B. Rate Formula 197

C. Occupancy Formulae 197

D. Death Rates 197

    1. General 197

    2. Surgical Death Rates 198

    3. Maternal/Fetal Death Rates 198

E. Autopsy Rates 198

F. Other Rates 199

G. Length of Stay 199

III. ANSWER KEY   **200**

References 211

INDEX   **212**

Preface

This textbook was designed and developed to provide health care students and professionals with a rudimentary understanding of the terms, definitions, and formulae used in computing health care statistics and to provide self-testing opportunities and applications of the statistical formulae. The primary emphasis is on inpatient health care data and statistical computations, but in most cases the applications can be transferred to the outpatient health care setting and other health care data as well.

Definitions, formulae, and terms are available in other books, but very few problems are included. The major weakness a teacher encounters when teaching students is not so much that they cannot manipulate a formula, but rather that they have difficulties in selecting the correct number to include in the formula. Skill in statistics is developed and accomplished through actual use of data and by answering problem-solving questions.

Although "statistics" is a term that creates a phobic state in some students, by working through problems, step by step, they can alleviate that fear. Students need only basic mathematical skills (addition, subtraction, multiplication, and division) to succeed in solving these problems. Self-tests are included after each new concept is introduced and a comprehensive test has been provided at the end of each chapter. This textbook has been developed so that students can evaluate their grasp of the material as they progress through each chapter.

The subject matter has been expanded to include basic statistical knowledge, such as measures of central tendency, frequency distributions, and graphing of representative data. There is also a preliminary chapter that reviews basic mathematical terms and concepts, such as rates, ratios, and proportions.

Some chapters include starred (*) questions followed by an R and a number, ie. *(R3). These questions are included as a review of previously presented material. The number indicates the text chapter in which the material was originally presented, to facilitate the review. Some faculty will choose to ignore these questions and others may want to include them.

This textbook was developed with the health information student in mind, but the material is applicable to all health care workers and students who are involved in allied health statistics and analysis. Written at a level that even the novice can read and understand, this textbook should be useful for students who have been afraid of or who have not understood statistical concepts.

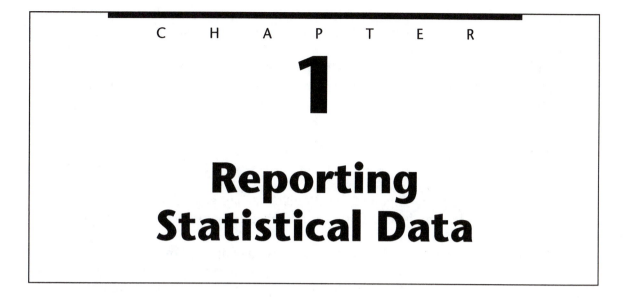

CHAPTER

1

Reporting Statistical Data

CHAPTER OUTLINE

A. Introduction
    1. Statistics and Data
    2. Scope of Book
B. Statistical Data Terms and Definitions
    1. Population vs. Sample
    2. Variable vs. Constant
    3. Qualitative vs. Quantitative Variables
    4. Discrete vs. Continuous Data
    5. Ungrouped vs. Grouped Data
    6. Descriptive vs. Inferential Statistics
C. Computerized Data
    1. Use
    2. Accuracy
D. Patient Data Collection
    1. Types of Data Collected
E. Abbreviations
    1. Patient Care
    2. Statistical
    3. Clinical Units
    4. Non-Official Abbreviations
F. Uses of Data
G. Summary
H. Chapter 1 Test

LEARNING OBJECTIVES

After studying this chapter the learner should be able to:

1. Define "statistics."
2. Define "data."
3. Distinguish clearly between:
    a. Population and sample.
    b. Variable and constant.
    c. Qualitative and quantitative data.
    d. Ungrouped and grouped data.
    e. Descriptive and inferential statistics.
4. Identify abbreviations used in health care statistics.
5. Describe various uses of data.

People are exposed daily to some type of statistical data or terms that is gathered and reported not only by the news media but also in the job arena. This is especially the case for those who work in the health care industry, where patient care data and statistics are compiled on a daily basis. Once we understand the meaningfulness of this data, we can become better managers and collectors of the data, thereby assuring appropriate uses for information.

A. INTRODUCTION

1. *Statistics and Data*

Statistics: A basic definition of statistics is "the mathematics of the collection, organization, and interpretation of numerical data, especially the analysis of population characteristics by inference from sampling."

Statistics is defined more broadly as a branch of applied mathematics, concerned with scientific methods for collecting, organizing, summarizing, and analyzing data. The term is frequently used to refer to recorded data, for example, reports that are issued regarding traffic accident statistics or the number of outpatients treated at an outpatient clinic. Statistics is also considered a branch of study that involves the theory, methodology, and mathematical calculation concerning the collection of various kinds of data.

Reasonable decisions and valid conclusions may be drawn based on the analysis of statistical data. Statistics therefore involves both numbers and the techniques and procedures to be followed in collecting, organizing, analyzing, interpreting, and presenting information in a numerical form.

Though the term statistics is a broad term, it is narrowed and defined by its representative data, such as accident statistics, hospital statistics, employment statistics, vital statistics, and several other descriptors.

Data: Data is defined as "information, especially information organized for analysis or used as the basis for a decision; numerical information." Data are those facts that any particular situation affords or gives to an observer. Some sources define data as raw facts and figures that are meaningless in and of themselves and refer to information as meaningful data—knowledge resulting from processing data.

The term data is generally and preferably the plural of the singular datum, though it is accepted in the singular construction as well. From this term references become more specific, for example, *data base* (also called *data bank*), which is a collection of data often arranged for ease and speed of retrieval. The preparation of information for processing by computers is referred to as *data processing*.

Enormous amounts of data and numbers are collected and tabulated daily in a hospital. A record is kept of most of the transactions that occur, including the number of patients admitted, the number of electrocardiograms performed, the number of babies born, the number of patients undergoing surgery, the number of patients who die, ad infinitum.

For this collected data to be useful and meaningful, various statistical methods and formulae must be applied.

Data are collected on inpatients, outpatients, emergency room patients, employees, and so on. Collected data must be compiled into a form that will have significance and that can be used to make comparisons for decision making.

2. Scope of Book

The purpose of this textbook is to introduce the reader to the terms, formulae, and computations used for hospital statistics, with the major emphasis on inpatient hospital statistics. Much of what applies to hospital inpatient statistics can be equally applied to outpatient data collection and statistical treatment of that data. As outpatient treatment has increased enormously during the past decade and as hospital inpatient admissions have declined, more and more data are handled daily, increasing the volume of numbers and data collected over a period of time—whether it be hourly, daily, weekly, monthly, quarterly, or yearly.

The major focus of this book is the statistical treatment of inpatient hospital statistics, with emphasis on definitions, formulae, and computations. It is to be assumed that the data referred to in this book are inpatient hospital data unless otherwise specified.

It is anticipated that the book's content and problems will be useful to hospital personnel whose function is the collection and interpretation of numerical data, especially health information personnel. Often the Health Information Department is the depository for medical information and the department is frequently responsible for compiling, collecting, and organizing data. This textbook provides material and problems to facilitate the processing and interpretation of these numerical data by the responsible personnel.

It should also be noted that those responsible for data collection should make sure to collect neither too much nor too little data. Data that are never used are not worth the added expense of collecting and processing them. In other words, cost effectiveness is achieved when the information is useful and of value to an individual or to a group.

B. STATISTICAL DATA TERMS AND DEFINITIONS

1. Population vs. Sample

Population: The term population refers to an entire group. A population is a set of persons (or objects) having a common observable characteristic.

Every ten years the United States Census Bureau conducts a census and sends census takers to each house and residence to count the number of inhabitants at each site throughout the United States. A hospital is also an example of a specific population—a group of people admitted for the purpose of receiving medical treatment and care. A population may also be comprised of all patients suffering from a specific disease or undergoing a specific form of treatment, such as radiotherapy.

Sample: A sample is a subset or small part of a population. Often information obtained from a sample is used to generalize from it to the entire population. For example, when checking the quality of an employee's work—for example, a transcriptionist—it is virtually unfeasible to check every word on every report transcribed by that transcriptionist during a designated week, month, or year. In such instances a sample is taken—say, two reports, or 5 percent of the transcribed reports—and the quality of the transcriptionist's work is based on this sample.

The majority of the data in this textbook will focus on population statistics, in which all the patients in a specific hospital will be referred to as the population. When handling information such as mortality (also referred to as death) statistics, census data, and pregnancy data, all cases will be included in the statistical treatment rather than every fifth case or tenth case, which makes use of sampling techniques. When employing sampling statistics, it is common to *infer* that this sample is representative of a given population (like an employee's work) and *deductions* are made relative to this sample. Probability analyses and deductive statistics will not be included in this textbook.

2. Variable vs. Constant

Variable: A variable is something that can change, in contrast to a constant, which remains the same.

Constant: A constant is something that assumes only one value; it is a value which is replaceable by one and only one number.

Variables are often expressed as symbols, such as X, x, Y, y, N, which can be replaced by a single number from a set of applicable numbers. Often it becomes desirable to compare variables and determine the relationship between them. For example, it may be useful to compare one variable, such as age, with another variable, such as occupation, or severity of illness, or a specific diagnosis.

A constant is a that which does not change and has one and only one value. A constant is one's date of birth or any value or specific that applies to everyone in the distribution.

3. Qualitative vs. Quantitative Variables

Qualitative Variables: Qualitative variables yield observations that can be categorized according to some characteristic or quality. Examples of this type of variable include a person's occupation, marital status, education level, race, etc.

Quantitative Variables: Quantitative variables yield observations that can be measured. Examples of this type of variable are height, weight, blood pressure, serum cholesterol, heart rate, etc. Quantitative data can be subdivided into discrete and continuous data.

4. Discrete vs. Continuous Data

Discrete Data: Discrete data are always expressed as a whole number or integer. This includes a specific numerical test score (for example, 80 out of a possible 100 points) or the number of red blood cells per cubic milliliter.

Continuous Variables: Continuous variables are those that fall into the category of "measured to the nearest." This includes data that in most instances would be measured in decimal fractions but are more commonly reported to the nearest whole number. Height, weight, and age are continuous variables. A person who is only two months away from her 22nd birthday is closer to age 22 than to age 21. A person measuring 5 feet 4 3/4 inches is closer to being 5 feet 5 inches than 5 feet 4 inches.

5. Ungrouped vs. Grouped Data

Ungrouped Data: Ungrouped data is a listing of all scores as they are obtained. Ungrouped data also refers to a distribution in which scores are ranked from highest to lowest or lowest to highest but each score has its own place in the array.

Grouped Data: Grouped data involves some type of grouping or combining of scores. The most common means of grouping is the counting or tallying of like scores. In this method, all identical scores are tallied and the number recorded after the score. If five pediatric patients were all admitted on the same day and two were 10 years of age, then two tally marks would be placed in the 10-year-old age column.

With a large range of scores, it often becomes necessary to combine some scores together and reduce the spread. Ages, even when recorded to the nearest whole number, would range from newborn to over 100 years of age. With a large number of scores, it becomes necessary to group and tally scores and thus narrow the range. Ages are often grouped, and may include a range by decade or some other grouping, say, newborn to 4 years; 5 years to 13 years; 14 to 21; 22 to 34; 35 to 49; 50 to 64; 65 to 79; 80 to 100.

6. Descriptive vs. Inferential Statistics

Descriptive Statistics: Descriptive statistics deal with data that are enumerated, organized, and possibly graphically represented. The decennial census carried out by the United States government is an example of descriptive statistics. The data gathered are obtained and then compiled into some type of table or graph.

Inferential Statistics: Inferential statistics are concerned with reaching conclusions. At times the information available is incomplete and generalizations are reached based on the data available. When generalizations about a population are made that are based on information obtained from a sample, inferential statistics are utilized. A common example relates to the inferences about a population that are based on opinion polls.

C. COMPUTERIZED DATA

1. Use

More and more data collections and computations are being carried out by computers, using both personal computers and on-line computers connected to a central mainframe. Local area networks (LANs) are increasingly being installed. As the size of a health care facility increases, the amount of data collected also increases and this collection is facilitated by computers. Even smaller institutions are finding it profitable to invest in computers that can be accessed at any time to print out the latest statistical information, such as the census, percent of occupancy, and other facts that management needs for decision making.

2. Accuracy

Accuracy is important when entering data either manually or by computer. Quality control measures should be incorporated to maintain correct data entry and accuracy. One should always ask whether the resultant figure from any computation is plausible and, if not, recheck the data entries.

D. PATIENT DATA COLLECTION

1. Types of Data Collected

Computerization in health care facilities has increased dramatically during the past decade and this trend will continue well into the future, making it easier to collect more data. The increased amount of information can be useful in decision making. The types of patient data that are collected in health care facilities can be classified into six broad categories, as follows:

a. *Dates*

Examples of dates included in this category are the patient's date of birth, date of admission, date of discharge, date of a surgical procedure, dates of various forms of treatment (both inpatient and outpatient), and date of delivery (giving birth).

b. *Counts*

Examples of counts include the number of patients admitted on a certain date or discharged on a certain date, the number of CBCs (complete blood count) performed or EKGs (electrocardiogram) or any number of other tests, the number of patients receiving physical therapy treatment or chemotherapy, the number of babies delivered live or aborted, the number of patients who died in the hospital or were treated in the emergency room.

c. *Test Results*

Laboratory tests are a major data collection component of inpatient and outpatient examinations. These include hematology tests such as CBC, WBC (white blood cell) differential, and RBC (red blood cell) morphology; blood chemistries such as blood glucose, BUN (blood urea nitrogen), and alkaline phosphatase; UA (urinalysis); CSF (cerebrospinal fluid) analysis; bone marrow tests; blood typing, serology, toxicology, and many more.

d. *Diagnoses*

Patients upon admission are assigned an admitting diagnosis (also called provisional or tentative diagnosis). Discharge diagnoses are assigned at the time of discharge and include the principal diagnosis and other diagnoses and complications. Each consultant who sees the patient provides diagnoses for their specialty area. Surgeons assign preoperative and postoperative diagnoses at the time of surgery. Diagnoses are assigned code numbers from which a disease and procedure index/data base are generated. Counts can be made for a specific disease to ascertain how many patients were diagnosed with that disorder in the period specified.

e. *Procedures*

If a patient undergoes a surgical procedure or diagnostic procedure, it is recorded, and most of these procedures are assigned code numbers as well. Totals can be generated for specific procedures (such as gastroscopies, mammographies, and hysterectomies) in a manner similar to that used for diagnoses.

f. *Treatment Outcomes and Assessments*

Upon discharge, a note is often written on a patient's medical record about the condition of the patient at the time of discharge and whether the patient was discharged home in good condition, transferred to another facility (nursing home, another hospital), or expired. Results of treatment can be recorded and various modalities of treatment can be compared based on these data. Treatment outcomes of one institution can also be compared with those of another and serve as the basis for research studies.

E. ABBREVIATIONS

Certain abbreviations are routinely used by hospitals with regard to data collection and analysis. Listed below, for easy reference, are some common abbreviations used throughout this text.

1. *Patient Care*

AMA	against medical advice	(patient left without a discharge order)
DOA	dead on arrival	
ER	emergency room	
IP	inpatient	
NB	newborn	
OB	obstetrical	
OP	outpatient	

2. *Statistical*

ADM	admission	(patient admitted to the hospital)
DIS	discharge	(patient discharged from the hospital)
A&D	admitted and discharged	(patient was admitted and discharged on the same day)

Also called *I&O* (in and out) in some facilities; others refer to such patients as "come and go." In this text they will be designated as A&D.

A&C   adults and children

This designation is used to refer to all patients other than newborns. It is used to separate patients into two categories—newborns and others. This designation is needed because many formulae require separate computations for the two groups—newborns vs. all other patients (A&Cs). The two populations have unique characteristics and need to be treated separately.

TRF-in	transferred in	(patient transferred into a clinical unit)
TRF-out	transferred out	(patient transferred out of a clinical unit)
>	greater than	
<	less than	
$\bar{c}$	with	(from the Latin word *cum*, meaning "with")
$\bar{s}$	without	(from the Latin word *sine*, meaning "without")
Σ	summation	(The uppercase Greek letter sigma means summation—it indicates that whatever follows the sign is to be added.)

3. *Clinical Units (Some of the More Common Designations)*

CCU	coronary care unit	NEURO	neurology/neurosurgery
ENT	ear-nose-throat	OB	obstetrics
ICU	intensive care unit	ONCO	oncology
MED	medical care unit	OPHTH	ophthalmology

ORTHO	orthopedics	REHAB	rehabilitation
PED	pediatrics	SURG	surgical care unit
PSYCH	psychiatry	UROL	urology

4. Non-Official Abbreviations

Throughout this text there will be abbreviations used which may not be used in all health care facilities but which facilitate computations that will be carried out in the various chapters of the text. Rather than stating the same words over and over, using an abbreviation facilitates brevity (or conciseness). Complete explanations describing each of these terms will be included in the chapters in which they are used. They are listed here for easy reference. For the sake of brevity, the following abbreviations will be used:

Cor	coroner/medical examiner case
CTT	census-taking time
DD	discharge days
DIPC	daily inpatient census
HP	hospital pathologist
IPSD	inpatient service day
LOS	length of stay

F. USES OF DATA

Data are used in a variety of ways, for example, to justify the opening or closing of clinical units in a hospital and to assess and justify the need for new equipment, facilities, and staff. Data are invaluable to physicians in determining the proper diagnosis and treatment of their patients. Data are also essential when assessing the quality of care administered by the hospital staff.

Quality assessment is a hospital-wide function. It applies not only to patient care but is also incorporated in other departments, such as patient accounts, housekeeping, and security and food service. Whether to validate the accuracy of an employee's work or to assess the quantity of work performed in a designated period of time, data serves as the primary means of performance evaluation. As health care costs keep rising and as patients are faced with higher co-payments and lower deductibles, patients will demand better quality for their medical dollars. As the crisis in health care continues, health care facilities will need quality data to justify expenditures and to demonstrate quality of care. A greater emphasis will be placed on quality assessment and improvement. TQM (total quality management) and CQI (continuous quality improvement) have been reverberating throughout health care facilities as well as manufacturing establishments. Data collected by the health care facility will become increasingly important in quality assessment and in demonstrating the need for facilities, staff, equipment, and services.

G. SUMMARY

1. Statistics is a broad term and makes use of data. Descriptive statistics and inferential statistics are representative types of statistics.

2. Data is information. Similar information gathered about a group becomes a data base. The processing of the information collected is referred to as data processing. Data terms include: discrete data, continuous data, grouped data, ungrouped data, and computerized data. A great variety of data can be collected, including dates, test results, diagnoses, procedures, and treatments.

3. A population includes an entire group. A sample is a subset of a population.

4. A variable is something that can change. A constant assumes only one value.

5. Variables are subdivided into qualitative and quantitative variables.

6. Abbreviations are used for the sake of brevity and are especially common in the health care arena. The abbreviations most commonly used in statistical computations are listed in this chapter.

7. Data has many uses and the proper collection and interpretation of data will become increasingly important as health care reimbursement dwindles and emphasis on quality assessment increases.

H. CHAPTER 1 TEST

1. Indicate whether the data represented in each of the following examples is part of a population or a sample:

   a. Twenty-five cases of TB have been reported in the past year and a patient care evaluation study is to be carried out using data from all 25 cases.   Population   Sample

   b. Sixty gastroscopies have been performed during the past two months and a study is to be carried out regarding various variables. Twenty-five of these cases will be reviewed.   Population   Sample

   c. Thirty-nine ER deaths were reported during the past year and the hospital administrator is requesting an analysis of all these deaths.   Population   Sample

2. Indicate the terms for:

   a. A value that can change   _____

   b. A value replaceable by only one number   _____

3. Indicate whether the following represent quantitative or qualitative variables:

   a. Number of days gestation   Quantitative   Qualitative
   b. Sex of patient   Quantitative   Qualitative
   c. Type of residence in which one resides   Quantitative   Qualitative
   d. Respiratory rate   Quantitative   Qualitative
   e. Blood pH   Quantitative   Qualitative
   f. Exercise engaged in for fitness   Quantitative   Qualitative
   g. Urinalysis glucose level   Quantitative   Qualitative
   h. Condition of patient at time of discharge   Quantitative   Qualitative

4. Indicate whether the data associated with the following are discrete or continuous:

   a. ESR (erythrocyte sedimentation rate)   Discrete   Continuous
   b. Height   Discrete   Continuous
   c. Blood glucose level   Discrete   Continuous
   d. Age   Discrete   Continuous
   e. Platelet count   Discrete   Continuous

f.   Deaths reported in November   Discrete   Continuous
g.   Minutes needed to walk a mile   Discrete   Continuous

5.   Grouping data: During the first two weeks in January, 48 adult patients were seen in surgical consultation. Their ages were recorded as follows:

58	73	91	18	27	55	33	21
59	65	77	42	48	63	28	47
39	49	62	37	81	84	72	66
44	55	80	27	37	77	59	56
61	51	47	58	73	48	49	38
77	80	56	66	59	88	67	73

a.   Rank the ages from oldest to youngest.

b.   List the score only once and place a tally mark after each score.

c.   Using the grouping below, place a tally mark after each interval:

94–97	66–69	38–41
90–93	62–65	34–37
86–89	58–61	30–33
82–85	54–57	26–29
78–81	50–53	22–25
74–77	46–49	18–21
70–73	42–45	

6.   Identify the following abbreviations:

a.   NB

b.   Σ

c.   A&D

d.   A&C

e.   DOA

f.   IP

g.   LOS

h.   ICU

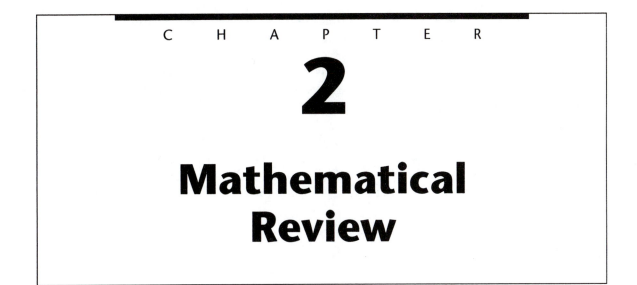

CHAPTER

2

Mathematical Review

CHAPTER OUTLINE

A. Fractions
    1. Numerator
    2. Denominator
    3. Quotient
B. Decimals
C. Percentages
D. Rates
E. Ratio
F. Proportion
G. Averaging

H. Rounding Data
I. Conversion to Another Form
    1. Fraction to Percentage
    2. Ratio to Percentage
    3. Decimal to Percentage
    4. Percentage to Decimal
    5. Percentage to Fraction
J. Computing with a Percentage
K. Summary
L. Chapter 2 Test

LEARNING OBJECTIVES

After studying this chapter the learner should be able to:

1. Explain the terms:
    a. Fraction
    b. Decimal
    c. Percentage
    d. Rate/Ratio/Proportion
2. Distinguish between the numerator and denominator of a fraction.
3. Average a set of numbers.

4. Round data to a specified number.
5. Convert a number from one form to another form, including:
    a. Fraction to percentage.
    b. Ratio to percentage.
    c. Decimal to percentage.
    d. Percentage to decimal.
    e. Percentage to fraction.

The use of the word data, as explained in the previous chapter, refers to numerical information and most commonly is information that has been organized in some way so that it can be analyzed and used as a basis for a decision. Once numbers have been collected, they are often arranged for ease and speed of retrieval. This is called a data base, a term heard frequently in a health care setting. Considerable data are compiled on both inpatients and outpatients, especially today when computers facilitate both the collection and arrangement of data.

The individual numbers gathered and collected on a patient become more meaningful when they are combined and compared with those of other patients, especially patients with similar conditions, ages, or other similarities. Data can be converted into usable information by using various mathematical and statistical formulae. This chapter reviews basic mathematical terms and computations needed to compute the rates and formulae in the chapters that follow.

A. FRACTIONS

Fraction: A fragment or part of a whole; small part; bit.

Example: If a pie is divided into six equal slices and an individual eats one slice, that individual has eaten one-sixth of the pie. If two slices of pie are eaten, one-third of the pie would be consumed (2/6 = 1/3). Three of the six slices being eaten results in half the pie being devoured (3/6 = 1/2).

Example: Substituting hospital data, if there are twelve beds set up and available on a clinical unit and eight of them are occupied by patients, then two-thirds (8/12 = 2/3) of the beds on that unit are filled but one-third (4/12 = 1/3) are still available.

SELF-TEST 1: Eighty-five babies are delivered during the month of May. Of these, 43 were born to a Caucasian female, 25 to an African American female, 12 to a Hispanic female, and five to an Oriental female. Indicate what fraction of these 85 babies was born to each race in May.

1. Numerator

Numerator: The top number (number above the line) of a fraction.

Example: In the fraction 6/16, 6 is the numerator.

SELF-TEST 2: Indicate the numerator for the following fractions:
   a. 3/13   b. 10/18   c. 6/5

2. Denominator

Denominator: The bottom number (number below the line) of a fraction.

Example: In the fraction 5/15, 15 is the denominator and 5 is the numerator.

SELF-TEST 3: Indicate the denominator for the following fractions:
   a. 7/17   b. 3/10   c. 9/8

3. Quotient

Quotient: The number resulting from division of one number by another. With fractions, the quotient is obtained by dividing the numerator by the denominator. The quotient is more correctly determined by dividing the dividend (numerator in a fraction) by the divisor (denominator of a fraction).

Example: Twenty cookies are to be divided among 15 people. To find how many cookies each person receives, 20 is divided by 15, resulting in a quotient of one-and-one-third cookies for each person (20/15).

SELF-TEST 4: Find the quotient for each of the following:

a. 100/45   b. 7/9   c. 18/25

B. DECIMALS

Decimal: An amount less than 1. A decimal is a fraction based on divisions that are powers to the negative base 10 (10 to the -1 power would be 1/10). (0.10 = 1/10; 0.01 = 1/100; 0.001 = 1/1000, etc.)

Example: If a pan of brownies is divided into ten pieces and eight are eaten, then 0.8 of the brownies in the pan were eaten (8/10 = 0.8).

Example: If ten residents of a city with a population of 10,000 are diagnosed with pertussis, then 0.001 have been afflicted.

SELF-TEST 5: What is the decimal equivalent of each of the following?

a. 5/100   b. 7/1000   c. 8/800

C. PERCENTAGES

Percentage: The number of times something happens out of every one hundred times. A percentage is a specific rate followed by a percent sign; it is a proportion of a whole.

Example: If 40 out of every 100 hospital employees have attained a four-year college degree, then it can be said that 40% of all employees at that hospital have earned a bachelor's degree.

SELF-TEST 6: Find the following percentages:

a. 6/100   c. 8/1000

b. 5/10   d. 56/100

D. RATES

Rate: Rate has many meanings. It can mean a value or price (as in 50 cents a pound); it can be a unit of something (as in the rate of speed is 30 mph, or the birthrate is 20 births per every 100 teenagers, or the interest rate is 8.6%). A rate is also a ratio, proportion, or rank. Most commonly a rate is expressed as a percentage.

Example: A bank advertises the interest rate for a savings account as 5%. A hospital reports an 85% occupancy rate. Statistics might show that the infection rate at a certain hospital during the previous year was 8%.

SELF-TEST 7: The newborn nursery reports that 120 infants were born at the hospital during the month of May. Five of these infants died shortly after birth and the rest were discharged. What is the newborn death rate?

E. RATIO

Ratio: A relationship between things or of one thing to another thing; it is also a rate or proportion. A ratio is generally expressed as a fraction (for example, 8/10 or 4/5). All rules that apply to fractions apply equally to ratios.

Ratios are also written with the numbers side-by-side and separated by a colon (8:10 or 4:5 or 65:100). The following are equivalent: 8/10; 4/5; 40/50; 80/100; 20:25; 12:15.

Example: Seven out of ten people admitted to the hospital are found to be over 50 years of age. This ratio could be written as 7/10 or 7:10.

SELF-TEST 8: One hundred operations were performed this past month. If 20 of these were orthopedic procedures, 12 were gynecological, 18 were ophthalmological, 22 were urological, and the remainder were general surgeries, what was the ratio for each surgical category?

F. PROPORTION

Proportion: A relationship of one portion to another or to the whole, or of one thing to another. A proportion is a ratio.

G. AVERAGING

Average: A number that represents a middle point between extremes. Statistically speaking, an average is referred to as a mean, or arithmetic mean, to distinguish it from the median and mode, which are also used statistically as measures of central tendency (see Chapter 10 for measures of central tendency).

Formula to Compute an Average: Add (summate) all scores in a distribution and divide by the number of scores in the distribution.

$$\text{Average} = \frac{\Sigma \text{ (Sum) of all scores}}{N} \qquad (N = \text{number of scores in the distribution})$$

Example: A student has taken ten math tests. The scores for these tests are: 100, 95, 85, 90, 78, 92, 87, 81, 72, 94. Summing the ten scores yields a total of 874. This total is then divided by 10 (number of tests taken), which results in an average math test score of 87.4 (or 87).

Example: A hospital's ten-day admission figures are reported as follows: 10, 15, 12, 8, 6, 18, 16, 5, 9, 13. To find the average number of patients admitted during this ten-day period, add all the admission figures (112) and divide by the number of days (10). The result is 11.2 (or 11), which indicates that during that period the hospital averaged eleven admissions per day.

SELF-TEST 9

1. The surgical center of a hospital lists the number of operations performed each day as follows: 6, 10, 8, 9, 5, 12, 7.

   Determine: Average number of operations performed each day during that week.

2. A hospital's yearly death records reveal the following monthly figures: 3, 4, 1, 2, 6, 2, 5, 8, 1, 4, 6, 3.

   Determine: Average number of deaths reported each month.

3. A total of 575 stress electrocardiograms were performed in May.

   Determine: Average number of stress EKGs performed daily in May.

4. A total of 1050 patients were seen in the ER during the first six months of a non-leap year.

   Determine: Average number of patients seen daily in the ER during the first six months of the year.

5. The following number of newborn babies were reported for the week: 2, 2, 4, 1, 3, 1, 3.

   Determine: Average number of babies born each day.

H. ROUNDING DATA

Why Round? When working with data, the result does not always compute to a whole number. When the scores in the previous section were averaged, the resultant average often included a decimal fraction. For instance, when averaging 9 + 10 the result comes to 9.5. In another instance, the number beyond the decimal point could continue indefinitely, as when averaging 6, 9, 7. Adding the three scores yields a total of 22 (6 + 9 + 7) and dividing by 3 results in an average score of 7.33333, etc., extending indefinitely. Often data must be rounded to a usable number.

Carried to. When dividing fractions, it is important to specify the decimal place to which the division should be carried out. It is generally better to carry out the division too far than not far enough. With the availability of hand-held calculators, the division can be carried out well beyond the place needed for most calculations. A division should be carried at least one place farther than the specified (*corrected*) decimal place for the final answer and rounded off to that specified place.

Corrected to. Once the quotient appears on the calculator display, it must often be shortened to an acceptable, specified length. Seldom are hospital data carried beyond two or three decimal places. When data are to be *corrected* to two decimal places, the calculation must be *carried* to three decimal places—at least one place beyond the requested place. If the answer is to be correct to the nearest whole number, it must be carried to one decimal place; if it is specified that the answer be correct to one decimal place it must be carried to two decimal places, and so on. This extra place is necessary to round the answer to the *correct* digit.

When to Increase or Round-up. If the last digit is five or greater, the preceding number should be increased one digit. If the last digit is less than five, the number remains the same. Be sure to note to what decimal place the computation should be "correct to" and then carry the answer one additional place and round the final answer, based on this additional digit.

Example: If 365.6 is to be rounded to the nearest whole number, the answer becomes 366 (since 0.6 is 0.5 or greater).

Example: If a computation results in an answer of 7.65 but the answer is to be "correct to" one decimal place, the answer becomes 7.7 (since the number following 6 is 5 or greater). (7.84 becomes 7.8.)

Example: If 17.655 is to be corrected to two decimal places, the answer becomes 17.66. (45.653 becomes 45.65.)

SELF-TEST 10

1. Round to the nearest whole number:

   a. 65.4
   b. 65.5
   c. 65.6
   d. 70.5
   e. 7051.4
   f. 0.6
   g. 38.499
   h. 595.85
   i. 148.475
   j. 10.05
   k. 15.555
   l. 55.505

2. Round correct to one decimal place:

   a. 12.35
   b. 27.625
   c. 31.6511
   d. 0.005
   e. 456.955
   f. 698.99
   g. 83.95
   h. 1.05
   i. 6.555
   j. 76.049

3. Round correct to two decimal places:

   a. 65.699
   b. 68.636
   c. 0.005
   d. 953.799
   e. 125.9995
   f. 65.666
   g. 17.999
   h. 79.995
   i. 100.055
   j. 1.1548

4. Round to the nearest

   a. hundred   3256
   b. tenth   5.781
   c. thousandth   0.0045
   d. hundredth   46.7385
   e. million   3,502,378
   f. ten   2184.73

g. hundredth   43.87500

h. thousand   45,679.88

$$\frac{\text{Numerator}}{\text{Denominator}} \times 100$$ (Add a percent sign to the result.)

I. CONVERSION TO ANOTHER FORM

1. *Fraction to Percentage*

Formula:

Example: To convert 60/80 to a percentage, divide 60 by 80, and then multiply the quotient by 100, which equals 75% [(60 ÷ 80) × 100 = 75].

Example: A test has five questions. A student answers two of the five correctly (2/5). Converting this to a percent, divide 2 by 5, and then multiply the quotient by 100, which gives a 40% score [(2 ÷ 5) × 100 = 40].

SELF-TEST 11: Convert the following fractions to percentages—correct to one decimal place.

a. 20/30   b. 25/50   c. 6/60

d. 32/78   e. 5/8

2. *Ratio to Percentage*

Formula: Convert ratio to fraction and proceed as in #1 above.

Example: One out of eight nurses indicated that he or she had worked a double shift the previous month. To convert this information to a percentage, divide 1 by 8, and then multiply the quotient by 100, which gives 12.5%, or 13% when rounded up [(1 ÷ 8) × 100 =12.5].

SELF-TEST 12: Convert the following ratios to a percent—correct to the nearest whole percent.

a. 1:3   b. 7:11   c. 5:6

d. 11:17   e. 15:60

3. *Decimal to Percentage*

Formula: Move decimal point *two* places to the right of the decimal point and add the percent sign.

Example: To convert 0.50 to a percentage, the decimal point is moved two places to the *right* (from 0.50 to 50.) and the number is followed by a percent sign (50%).

Example: Converting 0.001 to a percent, the decimal is moved two places to the right to give 0.1%. Note that since the answer is less than 1%, the decimal point remains even though it is moved two places to the right. ($0.001 = 1/1000 \times 100/1 = 1/10\%$ or 0.1%.) It is common practice to use a zero in front of a decimal point if the answer is less than 1; also zeros are eliminated to the right of the decimal point if they are not followed by another number. (50.100 becomes 50.1 or 50.1%.)

SELF-TEST 13

1. Convert the following decimals into percentages without rounding:
    a. 1.25   b. 0.635   c. 0.3

    d. 0.03   e. 0.006   f. 0.8235

    g. 0.0162   h. 0.55

2. Convert the following decimals into percentages, correct to the nearest whole number (no decimal).
    a. 3.25   b. 0.45677   c. 0.005

    d. 0.5555   e. 0.0166   f. 0.0449

4. Percentage to Decimal

Formula: Cross out the percent sign and move the decimal point two places to the *left* of the decimal point.

Example: To convert 65% to a decimal, eliminate the percent sign and move the decimal point from 65. to .65.

SELF-TEST 14: Convert the following percentages to a decimal:
a. 5%   c. 0.5%

b. 11.4%   d. 125%

5. Percentage to Fraction

Formula: Cross out percent sign and place the entire number (percentage) in the numerator and place 100 in the denominator.

Example: To change 55% to a fraction, eliminate the sign and place 55 in the numerator and 100 in the denominator.

Note: Fractions are often converted to their lowest form. In this example both 55 and 100 can be divided by 5, resulting in a fraction of 11/20, but either form is acceptable.

SELF-TEST 15: Convert the following percentages to the lowest fraction:
a. 75%   b. 87.5%   c. 33.33%

d. 112.5%   e. 20%   f. 84%

g. 50%   h. 98%

J. COMPUTING WITH A PERCENTAGE

When computing with a percentage, the percentage is converted to a decimal, as above, and used in that form.

Formula: Change percentage to decimal and multiply by N (total number in the distribution).

Example: If 60% of all patients admitted to the hospital have a blood glucose test, how many patients were administered a blood glucose test in the past year, out of 6000 admissions? Convert 60% to 0.60 and multiply by 6000 = 3600 patients.

Example: A hospital has 80% of its 120 beds filled. To find how many empty beds are present, change 80% to 0.80 and multiply by the number of beds (120 x 0.8 = 96 beds) and subtract from 120 (120 - 96 = 24). Alternatively, it can be said that if 80% of the beds are filled, 20% are empty. This 20% number can also be used for the computation (0.20 x 120 = 24 empty beds).

SELF-TEST 16

1. Convert 25% to the *lowest* fraction.

2. Convert 62.5% to the *lowest* fraction.

3. Convert 60% to the *lowest* ratio.

4. Convert 0.5% to a decimal.

5. Convert 3% to a decimal.

6. Convert 12% to a decimal.

7. A hospital reports that, in January, 40% of its patients had a blood glucose test. If there were 1050 patients in the hospital in January, how many had a blood glucose test?

8. If it is reported that two-thirds of all patients on a given day will have a CBC, how many out of every 100 patients will have a CBC? Correct your answer to the nearest whole number.

9. A medical records department has 28 full-time employees and 18% are home with the flu. How many employees are working?

10. A Salmonella outbreak occurs in a hospital and 8% of hospital-related people are diagnosed with the illness. If the hospital has 350 employees and the present patient count is 225, how many hospital-related people have been diagnosed with Salmonella—correct to the nearest whole number?

K. SUMMARY

1. A fraction is a part of a whole written as one number over another number. The numerator is the top number; the denominator is the bottom number. The quotient is obtained by dividing the top number by the bottom number.
2. A decimal is an amount less than one and is preceded by a decimal point; it is the fractional amount obtained by dividing the numerator by the denominator of a fraction.
3. A percentage is a decimal multiplied by 100; the percentage number is followed by a percent sign.
4. A rate is a quantity measured with respect to another measured quantity; it is often defined as the number of times something happens divided by the number of times it could happen.
5. A ratio (also known as a proportion) is the relationship between items or to other items.
6. An average is a measure of central tendency or relative proportion. To obtain the average for a distribution, the scores are summed and the total divided by the number of scores in the distribution.
7. Rounding is a common practice and specifies the number of places to which the computation should be carried out beyond the decimal point, rounding *up* if the final number is 5 or more.
8. Computations can be converted from one form to another—fraction, ratio, or decimal to percentage; percentage to fraction or decimal.
9. When computing with percentages, the percent is converted to a fraction or decimal before proceeding with the computation.

L. CHAPTER 2 TEST

1. Compute the following averages:
   a. Ten patients were discharged yesterday. Two patients were hospitalized three days, two were hospitalized four days, and the rest were in for 5, 7, 8, 1, 9, and 2 days, respectively. What was the average number of hospitalized days for this group, correct to one decimal place?

   b. During the past week, the following number of cases of measles were reported statewide each day: 7, 5, 12, 18, 22, 14, 9. What was the daily average, correct to one decimal place?

   c. A hospital reports the following number of autopsies performed each month by the hospital pathologist: 10, 9, 12, 12, 7, 14, 8, 11, 9, 11, 13, 7. What was the average number performed monthly, correct to the nearest whole number?

2. Round to two decimal places:
   a. 40.636   b. 40.666   c. 40.699

   d. 10.999   e. 18.555   f. 0.095

3. Round to the nearest whole number:
   a. 40.499   b. 70.555   c. 67.9

   d. 7770.4   e. 0.5   f. 55.5

4. Round to the nearest
   a. hundred   4455   e. hundredth   63.895

   b. tenth   4.657   f. ten   77.499

   c. thousandth   0.0055   g. thousand   87,485.7

   d. million   4,500,000

5. Convert to a percentage—correct to one decimal place:
   a. 60:80   b. 2/5   c. 0.03

   d. 0.66   e. 1.08   f. 7/8

   g. 6/50   h. 6:9

6. Convert to the lowest fraction:
   a. 60/100   b. 80%   c. 35/65

   d. 33/99   e. 10%   f. 5:100

7. Convert to a decimal—correct to two decimal places:
   a. 1/12   b. 2/15   c. 45/65

   d. 73%   e. 10:90   f. 4 out of 4

8. Compute the following—correct to the nearest whole number:
   a. If six out of ten patients admitted to the hospital are discharged in three days or less, how many out of 12,689 recorded admissions were hospitalized over three days?

   b. A hospital discharged 2895 patients in January. If three percent developed a hospital-based infection, how many were affected?

   c. A hospital reported 14,444 discharges during the past year. If 35 percent of these patients were seen in consultation, how many discharged patients were seen by a consultant?

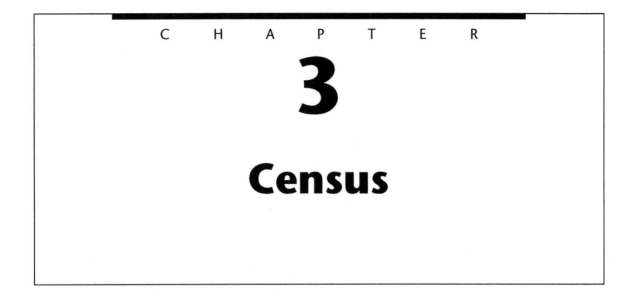

C H A P T E R

3

Census

CHAPTER OUTLINE

A. Census Collection and Terms
1. Census
2. Inpatient Census
3. Hospital Patients
4. Hospital Departments
5. Hospital Units vs. Services
6. Clinical Units
7. Census Taking
8. Admitted and Discharged the Same Day (A&D)
9. Daily Inpatient Census (DIPC)
10. Inpatient Service Day (IPSD)
11. Total Inpatient Service Days
12. Deaths/Discharges
13. Census Calculation Tips
14. Beds/Bassinets

B. Average Census
1. Average Daily Inpatient Census
2. Other Formulae for Census Averages
3. Example

C. Summary

D. Chapter 3 Test

LEARNING OBJECTIVES

After studying this chapter the learner should be able to:

1. Distinguish between
   a. Census, inpatient census, and daily inpatient census.
   b. Intrahospital transfer vs. interhospital transfer.
   c. A&C (adults and children) vs. NB (newborns).
   d. Clinical department vs. clinical unit vs. clinical service.
   e. Patients included in a bed count vs. bassinet count.

2. Define
   a. "IPSD" (inpatient service day).
   b. "A&D" (admitted and discharged).
   c. "Period" as used with regard to statistical computation.

3. Describe when a census is to be taken.

4. Identify deaths that are excluded from inpatient statistics.

5. Be able to compute
   a. Daily census.
   b. Period census.
   c. Average census.

The term *census* is familiar to the majority of the U.S. population because the U.S. Census Bureau takes a population census every ten years, at which time census takers go door-to-door to gather information regarding the number of people living at each residence. More than four-fifths of the world's population is counted in some kind of census. Facilities of all types—including hospitals, nursing homes, homeless shelters, day care centers, and so forth—enumerate census data. This data is kept daily, weekly, monthly, and for other specified intervals.

A. CENSUS COLLECTION AND TERMS

1. Census

The *American Heritage Dictionary* defines census as "an official, usually periodic enumeration of population." A census is a count—a count of people. This count can be of the population as a whole or a subgroup such as a hospital or even a clinical unit within a hospital.

2. Inpatient Census

The *Glossary of Health Care Terms* defines inpatient census as "the number of inpatients present at any one time."

3. Hospital Patients

A hospital provides examinations and treatments for patients in several different categories. The two major categories are (a) inpatients and (b) outpatients (also referred to as ambulatory care patients). Statistics are compiled separately on patients in these two categories.

a. Inpatients

A hospital inpatient is a patient who has been formally admitted to the hospital and to whom room, board, and continuous nursing service is provided in an area of the hospital where patients generally stay at least overnight. Inpatients (IP) are admitted to the hospital and assigned a hospital bed on a clinical unit.

Patients admitted to nursing homes (extended care facilities) are nursing home inpatients, and inpatient statistics are compiled on these patients in their respective facility. Nursing homes are subdivided into skilled nursing facilities, intermediate care facilities, and residential care facilities. Some nursing homes provide two or more of these types of care. (Please refer to the *Glossary of Health Care Terms* which is listed in the References section, or some other reference source for an explanation of these terms.)

b. Outpatients

Outpatients (OP) receive service on a more limited basis and are not assigned an inpatient hospital bed. A hospital outpatient is defined as a hospital patient who receives services in one or more of the facilities of the hospital when not currently an inpatient or a home care patient. Another term used to describe patients who are not considered inpatients is home care patients (those to whom care is provided in their place of residence).

Outpatient admissions usually are for laboratory tests [CBC, chemistry profile, GTT (glucose tolerance test), lipid profile], x-rays, physical therapy, and even outpatient surgery. These data are recorded separately to evaluate services received by patients and services rendered by the health care facility.

4. Hospital Departments

A hospital consists of many departments that provide a wide range of services to patients. A few of the typical hospital departments are health information, patient accounts, clinical laboratory, radiology, physical medicine and rehabilitation (PM&R), and outpatient surgery.

5. Hospital Units vs. Services

The words "service" and "unit" are often misused. A unit or division is an organizational entity, such as an inpatient unit or, even more specifically, a medical care unit, surgical unit, or special care unit such as ICU (intensive care unit) or drug dependency unit. Smaller hospitals generally have fewer administrative units than larger hospitals. The most common units are medical, surgical, obstetrics, newborn, and pediatrics.

The *Glossary of Health Care Terms* defines medical services as "the activities related to medical care performed by physicians, nurses, and other health care professional and technical personnel under the direction of a physician." It covers any medically related care (medical or surgical) provided to a patient by a member of the health care team. It ranges from blood drawn for a laboratory test to range of motion (ROM) exercises administered by a physical therapist to open heart surgery for a heart transplant.

A medical staff unit may be serviced by many medical staff specialties. Patients may be under the care of internists, gastroenterologists, cardiologists, oncologists, neurologists, or any number of other specialists. Age may also be a factor, with separate units designated for newborns and pediatric patients.

6. Clinical Units

Hospital beds are arranged into groupings called hospital units or clinical units or nursing units. These units are then staffed with nurses and other appropriate hospital personnel and are distinguished from one another by the type of cases primarily being treated—medical, surgical, orthopedics, pediatrics, etc.—or by their location, such as 3 North, 4 East, or 2B, 1A, etc., or by an abbreviation of the name of the type of care provided on that unit—for example, NB, OB, GYN, ORTHO, or PSYCH.

7. Census Taking

Census taking is the process of counting patients. Each day a hospital keeps track of the number of patients treated both as inpatients (IPs) and outpatients (OPs) and the services administered to patients. Throughout this book the census applications will apply to inpatients, but some of these statistics can also be applied to outpatient data.

a. Time of Day

The most important factor is *consistency*. A hospital needs to establish the time of day when all nursing units will take and report the census and this must be consistent every day and on all units. Usually midnight is chosen as "census-taking time" (CTT), because this is a time of day when activity has usually decreased, compared to the busier times of the day. However, if another time should be selected, it should be adhered to every day and on all nursing units.

b. *Reporting*

A designated person on each unit counts the patients present (on units) at the designated "census-taking time" (CTT). All patients must be accounted for. A hospital establishes a form for recording the census that includes a listing of patients admitted since the last census was taken, the patients discharged since the previous census, the patients who died in the past 24-hour period, and the patients who were transferred—either transferred-in (TRF-in) to the unit from another nursing unit in the hospital or transferred-out (TRF-out) to another nursing unit.

Example: Mary Jones is a patient on the medical unit and is taken to surgery at 8 A.M. Following surgery Mary is transferred to the surgical unit. Mary would be listed as a TRF-out on the census for the medical unit and as a TRF-in on the census for the surgical unit.

c. *Central Collection*

The data that is collected on each unit then has to be sent to a central collection area so that the hospital census can be established. This central area may be nursing service, administration, admitting, the health information department, or any other centralized reporting area. It is the responsibility of this designated area to make sure that the data is correct, that it corresponds to the total daily admissions and discharges, and that the inclusive intrahospital totals of transferred patients be equal—that is, that the total of all patients transferred in (TRF-in) to units equals the total of those transferred out (TRF-out).

d. *Transfers*

1) *Types of Transfers*

   a) INTRAHOSPITAL TRANSFERS

   Intrahospital transfers are transfers within a health care facility from one clinical unit to another clinical unit within the same facility. The prefix *intra* means "within" and thus these are the transfers from one nursing unit to another. (If Sue Smith is transferred out of one nursing unit, she would have to be transferred in to another unit unless she was discharged.) Thus the *total* intrahospital TRF-ins would always have to equal the intrahospital TRF-outs. If there is a discrepancy, the central collection area must play detective to find out where the mistake occurred.

   Note: The TRF-in and TRF-out totals on one specific clinical unit may not be equal because a unit may receive more than they lose or vice versa, but the *total* within a hospital (all units combined) must be equal.

   b) INTERHOSPITAL TRANSFERS

   Interhospital transfers are transfers to another hospital (the prefix *inter* means "between"). Since these patients will no longer be cared for at the hospital, they are discharged and will be listed on the census form as a discharge rather than as a transfer. However, hospitals often record on the face sheet where the patient went at the time of discharge—such as home, transferred to a nursing home, transferred to another hospital— and the name of the hospital or nursing home to which the patient was transferred.

2) *Counting Transfers*

A transfer is counted as a census patient only on the unit on which the patient is present at census-taking time (CTT).

Example: The following occurred on March 1. Sally Smith was admitted to the medical unit. It was found that she needed emergency surgery and she was taken to surgery, from which she was transferred to the surgical unit. Her condition worsened and she was transferred to ICU. There her condition stabilized and she was transferred back to the surgical unit. Where will Sally be counted at the end of the day at the census-taking time? Sally will be listed as a TRF-out on the medical unit; TRF-in to the surgical unit as well as TRF-out of the surgical unit; TRF-in and TRF-out of ICU; and again listed as TRF-in on the surgical unit, where she is counted as an inpatient for the March 1 census report at the CTT.

Note: A patient may only be counted as present on *one* unit even though the patient may have been on other units at different times of the day.

8. Admitted and Discharged (A&D)

The abbreviation A&D represents patients who are admitted and discharged on the same day. These patients are not to be confused with OPs, who are also admitted and discharged on the same day but are not considered inpatients. Remember that an IP is assigned an inpatient hospital number and is admitted to a hospital bed (called a bed count bed) and receives all the services accorded an inpatient. With the increase in outpatient treatment and services for many conditions that formerly required inpatient care, this term can be confusing. The number of A&D patients will generally be small, but there will be some who die, some who are transferred to another hospital, and even some who leave against medical advice, all of whom could fall into this A&D category. Since they have been treated and given service at your hospital, they will need to be included in the census.

9. Daily Inpatient Census (DIPC)

The term daily inpatient census refers to the number of inpatients present at the census-taking time each day *plus* any inpatients who were admitted and discharged (A&D) after the census-taking time the previous day.

A patient admitted after the census was taken (say, midnight of March 2) and before the census was taken the following day (March 3) would not be counted in the March 3 census because the patient was no longer present at CTT. However, the patient had received service in the hospital as an inpatient on March 3 even though the patient is no longer present at CTT. This patient is an A&D and will be included in the Daily Inpatient Census. For example, if Mary Morse is admitted at 8 A.M. on March 2 and discharged at 10 P.M. the same day, Mary will no longer be in the hospital at CTT but she did receive service on March 2, service for which the hospital should be credited. Thus, the Daily Inpatient Census (DIPC) is the census total (March 2 in this example) *plus* any A&Ds for that date (such as Mary Morse, who was an A&D on March 2).

10. Inpatient Service Day (IPSD)

An inpatient service day is a unit of measure denoting the services received by *one* inpatient during *one* 24-hour period.

The 24-hour period is the 24 hours between census-taking times. Assuming midnight is the CTT, any patient who received inpatient service during that 24-hour period counts as one inpatient service day. Other terms occasionally used for inpatient service day are "patient day," "inpatient day," "census day," or "bed occupancy day"—with inpatient service day the preferred term. The term inpatient service day includes not only a patient present at census-taking time but also a patient admitted and discharged the same day.

An inpatient service day total is the sum all inpatients who received service on a specific day. Each inpatient receiving service on a specific date is recorded as one inpatient service day and the total of all inpatients receiving service on that date is the inpatient service day total for that date. Based on these definitions, it is seen that the Daily Inpatient Census (DIPC) and Inpatient Service Day total (IPSD) compilations will be identical. Remember that these are daily figures—totals for one specific day.

a. **Unit of Measure vs. Totals**

  1) *Unit of Measure*

   A unit is the smallest amount to be measured, and in the statistical reporting to follow, a "unit" is represented by the singular term "day" as opposed to the plural "days," which is a total of the individual units. Each individual patient is credited with an inpatient service day for service in the hospital on a certain date. As previously mentioned, this includes a patient present at census-taking time (CTT) as well as a patient admitted and discharged (A&D) the same day.

  2) *Totals*

   Units of measure get combined into totals that are used for statistical purposes. Each patient is one "unit," but it is important to know the total amount of service rendered on a particular day or for a specific period of time. For instance, if 150 patients received service in the hospital on a specific date (say June 3) there would be a total of 150 inpatient service *days* for June 3. Note the use of the plural *days* as compared to the use of *day* for a unit designation. Also, it is important to know how many patients were given service for a certain period of time, which could include weeks, months, or even years. We may need to compare one year's totals with those of the previous year or compare last month's data with this month's, and so on. The period to be totaled is specified and all the inpatient service days will be added together to get the total.

b. *Period*

  Any combination of days will make up a period. A period may be two days; it may be one week or two weeks; it may be a month, half-month, two months; it may be a year, half-year, five years.

c. *Synonymous Figures*

  The value for Daily Inpatient Census (DIPC) and Inpatient Service Days (IPSD) will be identical. Both terms incorporate the same data—census-taking time (CTT) total plus inpatients admitted and discharged the same day (A&Ds). Whenever hospital statistics are computed, the DIPC or IPSD totals are used rather than census (CTT) totals because they are more representative of service rendered by the hospital.

d. **Watch Out**

Do not confuse the terms
Census/Inpatient Census *with*
Inpatient Service Day/Daily Inpatient Census (IPSD/DIPC)

The terms census or inpatient census are only counts at CTT. They *do not* include inpatients admitted and discharged the same day. The terms Inpatient Service Day (IPSD) or Daily Inpatient Census (DIPC) include the A&Ds as well as inpatients present at the time of the census count.

11. Total Inpatient Service Days

Total inpatient service days refers to the sum of all inpatient service days for each of the days in the period under consideration.

a. **Daily Recording—Recording of Daily Inpatient Census (DIPC) and Inpatient Service Days (IPSD)**

The beginning census is the census taken at census-taking time the previous day. To this number one patient day is *added* for each admission. Also, one patient day is *subtracted* for each discharge that occurred during that day (during the 24 hours following the previous census). Transferred-ins (TRF-in) are *added* to the subtotal and transferred-outs (TRF-out) are *subtracted*. (*Note*: Hospital-wide, the TRF-ins will equal the TRF-outs, but in computing unit totals these will not necessarily be identical.) Then, to this subtotal, one inpatient day must be *added* for each patient who was both admitted and discharged (A&Ds) between the two successive census-taking hours. This final total, then, is most representative of the amount of service rendered by the hospital on that specific day.

b. **Example**

For illustrative purposes, let us say that 155 inpatients were present at CTT on June 1. Fifteen patients were admitted to the hospital as inpatients on June 2. Five inpatients were transferred-out of a clinical unit and transferred-in to another clinical unit on June 2. Eight inpatients were discharged on June 2 (before CTT). Two patients were admitted and discharged the same day.

Solution: Record the June 1 census (155); *add* the admissions (15); *subtract* the discharges (8); *add* the TRF-ins and *subtract* the TRF-outs (both should be equal and cancel out); *add* the A&Ds (2). A total of 164 inpatients received service on June 2 (155 + 15 - 8 + 2 = 164).

12. Deaths/Discharges

a. **Included**

Deaths are considered discharges and, although they are recorded separately, they are included in the total discharges *unless* the term *live* discharges is used. In this latter instance, the deaths must be added to the live discharges to get the total number of inpatient discharges. Thus the word "discharges" includes deaths and live discharges.

b. Not Included

1) *Fetal Death*

A fetus that was not alive at the time of delivery was never a patient and is *not* included in inpatient hospital statistics. It is recorded and included only in specific formulae with the word "fetal" in them—fetal death rate and fetal autopsy rate. The term "stillborn" is still in use (though fetal death is preferred) in some facilities. A stillborn infant is classified as a fetal death.

2) *DOA*

The abbreviation DOA stands for Dead on Arrival. As pointed out earlier, a patient who is brought to the hospital with no signs of life and is never revived was never an inpatient and therefore is not included in inpatient census data.

3) *OP Death*

Only inpatients are included in inpatient hospital statistics. Outpatient data are maintained separately. An outpatient death would be recorded as part of the outpatient data. Remember that a patient must have been alive on admission to be considered an inpatient and be assigned an inpatient hospital bed.

13. Census Calculation Tips

In figuring census data, it is often helpful to use plus (+) signs and minus (-) signs in front of data to indicate whether a number should be added or subtracted from other numbers. Also, crossing out or drawing a line through data that are not relevant may also be helpful.

Example: Orthodedic ward—

		Statistic	Applying Hint
May 31	Midnight census	43	+ 43
June 1	Admitted	8	+ 8
	Discharged	2	- 2
	TRF-in	1	+ 1
	TRF-out	0	
	24-hour patients (A&D)	2	x (not counted)

Question 1. What is the census for June 1?

Solution: Placing a plus or minus in front of data helps identify which numbers to *add* and which to *subtract*, and, by lightly crossing out the two A&Ds, we indicate these are not to be included in the census. (Remember that the term "census" means the count at CTT and that A&Ds are *not* included in the census).

Answer: 50 (43 + 8 - 2 + 1 = 50)

Question 2. What is the Daily Inpatient Census for June 1?

Solution: The DIPC includes A&Ds and therefore the two A&Ds excluded above are included here. Thus, a plus 2 (+2) is added to the above total.

Answer: 52 (43 + 8 - 2 + 1 + 2 = 52) or (50 + 2 = 52)

Question 3. What is the Inpatient Service Day figure for June 1?

Solution: Since this value is identical to that for Daily Inpatient Census, the A&Ds are included and added as above.

Answer: 52 (See computation in Question 2.)

14. Beds/Bassinets

a. Inpatient Classification Categories

The two categories into which hospital inpatients are most commonly placed are

1. Adults and Children (A&C)
2. Newborn (NB)

b. Beds

Hospitalized patients are assigned to either a bed or a bassinet for statistical purposes. Hospitals are also set up and staffed for a certain number of beds and bassinets. Counts are conducted daily to find out how many of these beds and bassinets are being used.

Bed Statistics include all patients who are *not* born in the hospital during that hospitalization. Inpatients admitted to an inpatient hospital bed are included in the category designated as "Adults and Children" (A&C). The majority of the A&Cs are exactly what the term describes and they occupy an inpatient hospital bed. However, babies born on the way to the hospital or at home and then admitted are assigned one of these so-called "beds" even though they are placed in a bassinet or isolette. This is done to evaluate services between the two levels of care.

c. Bassinets

Only babies born in the hospital are included in the category referred to as "Newborns" (NB). These are the babies included in "bassinet" statistics. Remember that babies born at home or en route to the hospital are not included in the newborn bassinet census even though they are admitted shortly after birth. The infants in this latter category are assigned a so-called "bed" and are not included in the bassinet census statistics.

d. Adults and Children (A&C)

This category includes any inpatient admitted to the hospital other than a newborn born in the hospital. When census data are recorded, the data for adults and children are kept separate from that of newborns. When just the word "inpatient census" or "inpatient service days" is used, it refers to the adults and children census data.

e. Newborns (NB)

Any infant born in the hospital is considered a newborn and is included in the bassinet count and the newborn data statistics. Since the care required by these patients is quite different from that required by adults and children, the two groups are kept separate for statistical reporting and comparisons.

SELF-TEST 17

1. Hospital census on May 3 is 456.

    On May 4:   Admissions   58

    Discharges   45

    A&D   6

    DOA   3

    Calculate:

    a. Census for May 4.

    b. Daily inpatient census (DIPC) for May 4.

    c. Inpatient service day (IPSD) figure for May 4.

2. Newborn nursery census for May 1 = 22

    On May 2:   Births   4

    Discharges   2

    Fetal deaths   2

    TRF-in   0

    TRF-out   1

    Calculate: Census for May 2.

3. A hospital has a total of 100 patients at midnight (CTT) on July 1. On July 2 two patients are admitted in the morning and discharged in the afternoon. Another patient is admitted at noon but expires at 4:30 that same afternoon. A patient who was admitted two days ago is transferred to another hospital on July 2. No other patients are admitted or discharged on July 2.

    Calculate:

    a. Inpatient census for July 2.

    b. Daily inpatient census for July 2.

    c. Inpatient service day figure for July 2.

4. August 1—Inpatient census at midnight (CTT) = 150

August 2:	A. Adams	admitted	8 A.M.		
	B. Barnes	admitted	9 A.M.		
	C. Carlson	admitted	10 A.M.	discharged	6:00 P.M.
	D. Doran			discharged	3:30 P.M.
	E. Edwards			expired	11:15 A.M.
	F. Foster	admitted	1 P.M.		
	G. Foster	(NB—born at 8:45 P.M.)			
	H. Horn	DOA			

Calculate:

a. Inpatient census for August 2.

b. Daily inpatient census for August 2.

c. Inpatient service day figure for August 2.

5. The following inpatient service day figures are recorded for the month of April at Holy Family Hospital, a 50-bed hospital.

April	1	45	April	11	35	April	21	44
	2	30		12	41		22	48
	3	35		13	47		23	35
	4	25		14	48		24	36
	5	47		15	49		25	38
	6	48		16	50		26	42
	7	38		17	40		27	44
	8	42		18	41		28	40
	9	43		19	43		29	52
	10	36		20	47		30	41

Calculate:

a. Inpatient service day total for April.

b. Inpatient service day value for April 20.

c. Inpatient service day total for April 7 through April 15.

d. Average daily inpatient census for April.

B. AVERAGE CENSUS

1. *Average Daily Inpatient Census (Average Daily Census)*

Average number of inpatients present each day for a given period of time.

Formula:

$$\frac{\text{Total inpatient service days for a period}}{\text{Total number of days in the period}}$$

a. *Explanation*

Average figures are often more representative than totals for a given period of time and, even though there are periods when a large number of patients are serviced, there may also be periods when the reverse is true. Evaluating census data is easier when comparing the average daily inpatient census rather than comparing daily census totals.

b. *Separate A&C/NB Data*

Since census data for adults and children and for newborns were recorded separately, the averages are also figured on the respective individual data bases rather than combined into one figure. Since finding an average involves dividing by the number of days in a period, that period will again need to be specified—for example, a week, month, three months, six months, or a year.

c. *Days in Month*

For computing averages, one needs to know how many days there are in each month. There are several methods for remembering this, including:

Jingle. Thirty days hath September, April, June, and November. All the rest have 31, save February, which has 28 in line and leap year makes it 29.

Knuckles. Make a fist with both hands, keeping the thumbs hidden. Start at the little finger side of either hand and begin with January, pointing to the top knuckle (MCP joint). Then name the months by pointing first to the knuckle and then to the depression between the knuckles. If the month lands on a knuckle, the month has 31 days. If it falls in a depression, it has either 28 or 30 days (any month except February would have 30 days).

d. *Leap Year*

To determine whether a year is a leap year, divide the year by 4 and, if the quotient is a whole number without a remainder, the year is a leap year. For instance, 1988 divided by 4 results in a quotient of 497 with no remainder, indicating 1988 was a leap year. However, if 1986 is divided by 4, the result is 496 with a remainder of 2; thus 1986 was not a leap year and had only 28 days in February rather than 29.

e. *Rounding*

When dividing numbers, the quotient does not always turn out to be a whole number, and therefore the rules for rounding will need to be followed. When the figures are large, it is usually adequate to carry out the answer to two decimal places and round the answer correct to one decimal place. Sometimes the results are also recorded correct to the nearest whole number.

f. *Logical Answers*

Whenever decimal points or percentages are involved, it is very important to watch the placement of a decimal point. Obviously, there is a great difference between 2.10, 21.0, and 210. Many errors can be averted by asking yourself if the answer makes sense. If you work at a 210-bed hospital and the average inpatient service days for the month of January are reported as 20.1, the answer is most probably incorrect because an average this low would probably jeopardize a hospital's existence and possibly lead to its demise. A result of 2010 is also absurd and therefore impossible. Thus, it is extremely important to watch decimal points and to ask yourself if the answer is logical.

2. *Other Formulae for Census Averages*

a. *A&C*

Formula: Adult and Children Average Daily Inpatient Census (or) Average Daily Inpatient Census Excluding Newborns:

$$\frac{\text{Total inpatient service days (excluding newborns) for a period}}{\text{Total number of days in the period}}$$

b. **NB**

Formula: Average Daily Newborn Inpatient Census

$$\frac{\text{Total newborn inpatient service days for a period}}{\text{Total number of days in the period}}$$

c. **Clinical Unit**

Formula: Average Daily Census for a Clinical Unit

$$\frac{\text{Total IP service days for the clinical care unit for a period}}{\text{Total number of days in the period}}$$

3. **Example**

In Question #5 on the Self-Test in the previous section (Holy Family Hospital with 50 beds), a total of 1250 inpatient service days were recorded for the month of April. To compute the average daily inpatient census for the month of April, one would take the 1250 IPSD total and divide by the 30 days in the month of April, which results in an average daily inpatient census of 41.7 patients for the month of April for the 50-bed hospital.

SELF-TEST 18

1. St. Phillip's Hospital records the following:

	IP Service Days	Bed Count
January through April	43,725	400
May through August	59,218	500
September through December	65,383	550

Calculate: Average daily inpatient census for each of the three periods.

2. A 250-bed hospital with 20 newborn bassinets records the following inpatient service days for the month of March:

A&C: 7380

NB: 558

Calculate:

a. Average daily combined inpatient census.

b. Average daily adults and children census.

c. Average daily newborn census.

3. A hospital reported the following statistics for September:

Counts	Beds = 150	Bassinets = 15
Census (midnight of August 31)	A&C = 140	NB = 11
Admissions	A&C = 310	NB = 90
Discharges (live)	A&C = 300	NB = 92
Deaths	A&C = 15	NB = 2
Fetal deaths: 5		
Inpatient service days	A&C = 4236	NB = 410

Calculate:

a. Inpatient census for midnight of September 30.

b. Average daily inpatient census for September.

c. Average daily newborn census for September.

4. The following information is reported for three clinical units during the month of November:

	Pediatrics	Orthopedics	Psychiatric
Bed Count	12	15	10
Beginning census	10	12	6
Admissions	85	122	54
Discharges (live)	86	120	53
Deaths	1	3	0
Inpatient service days	344	433	284

Calculate:

a. Average daily inpatient census for each of the three clinical units.

b. Ending census (November 30) for each of the three clinical units.

c. Total inpatient service days for the three clinical units for the month of November.

C. SUMMARY

1. *Keep A&C Data Separate from NB Data*
   Census counts are occasionally combined, but IPSD totals are generally kept separate to facilitate statistical computations.
2. *Census/Inpatient Census*
   a. To determine: Count patients remaining at the census-taking time (CTT).
      1) Count is taken on the clinical units.
      2) Clinical units send their count to a central collecting department.

3) Intrahospital transfers are recorded.
Record is kept of patients transferred-in (TRF-in) and transferred-out (TRF-out). Transfers present on the unit at CTT are counted.
4) A&Ds are *not* counted in a census or inpatient census.
   b. *DIPC/IPSD*
   Count patients present at CTT and add A&Ds. (Add to the census [#1 above] the A&Ds for that day.)
   c. *Total IPSD for the Period*
   Add IPSD figure for each day in the designated period. (Be sure to use IPSD figures rather than census figures.)
   d. *Average Daily Inpatient Census (DIPC)*
   Total the IPSD for the period and divide by the number of days in the period.
   1) Figure A&C and NB averages separately.
   2) Divide by the number of days in the period.
   3) Apply the same rules to determine the average DIPC for a clinical unit.

D. CHAPTER 3 TEST

Note: All calculations should be carried out correct to one decimal place.

1. Distinguish between "daily inpatient census" (DIPC) and inpatient census.

2. To find the average daily inpatient census, what is placed in the denominator?

3. When must a census be taken?

4. Must TRF-ins equal TRF-outs on a daily census report—

   a. on individual clinical units?

   b. hospital-wide (total from all units combined)?l

5. A patient admitted to Unit A is transferred to Unit B the same day. On which unit is the patient counted at CTT?

6. When would a newborn (NB) be considered an A&D?

Note: For the remaining questions assume that the CTT is midnight.

7. Applegate Hospital records the following:

		A&C	NB	Other
May 31:	Census	141	10	
June 1:	Admissions	8	3	
	Discharged live	2	2	
	Deaths	1	0	
	Fetal deaths			2
	DOAs			2
	A&D	2	0	

Calculate:

a. Census for June 1.

b. IP census for June 1.

c. DIPC for June 1.

d. IPSD for June 1.

8. Three clinical units recorded the following information for April:

	Urology	*ENT*	*Ophth*
Bed count	18	16	24
Beginning census	15	12	20
Admissions	62	51	89
Discharges (live)	59	48	86
Deaths	1	0	1
IPSD	501	418	607

Calculate:

a. Census for April 30 for each clinical unit.

b. IPSD total for the three units combined for April.

c. Average DIPC for each unit for April.

9. A 65-bed hospital recorded the following data for May.

		IPSD			*IPSD*			*IPSD*
May	1	50	May	11	48	May	21	55
	2	50		12	56		22	58
	3	49		13	58		23	62
	4	54		14	56		24	65
	5	52		15	59		25	63
	6	51		16	60		26	62
	7	50		17	59		27	60
	8	43		18	58		28	60
	9	44		19	54		29	62
	10	46		20	55		30	63
							31	50

Calculate:

a. IPSD for May 20.

b. IPSD total for May 21 through May 31.

c. Average DIPC for May 21 through May 31.

d. Total IPSD for the month of May.

e. Average IPSD for the month of May.

10. Jan 31:   Census   456
    Feb 1:   Admissions   58
                 Discharges   45
                 A&D   6
                 DOA   3

Calculate:

a.   Census for February 1.

b.   IPSD total for February 1.

c.   DIPC for February 1.

11. A newborn unit reports the following:

    Bassinet count   21
    Last census   15
    Births   5
    Fetal deaths   2
    TRF-in   0
    TRF-out   1

Calculate: Census at CTT.

12. St. Peter's Hospital reports:

    A&C admissions for the year   998
    A&C discharges for the year   989
    A&C IPSD for the year   36,440

    Calculate: Average A&C daily inpatient census for the year.

13. An 18-bed surgical unit reports the following:

    Patients remaining at midnight 12
    Next day—Admissions   4
            Discharges   3
            TRF-in   2
            TRF-out   0
            A&D   2

    Calculate: Census at CTT.

14. Day 1: Census   125
    Day 2: Admissions   8
           Discharged live   4
           Deaths   2
           A&D   2

Calculate:

a. Ending census on day 2.

b. DIPC for day 2.

c. IPSD total for day 2.

15. May 31:   Census   150

    June 1:

ADM/DIS	Time Admitted	Time Discharged
A. Adams	8:00 A.M.	4:50 P.M.
B. Brown	9:00 A.M.	
C. Carson	10:18 A.M.	
D. Davis		11:55 A.M.
E. Edwards	2.40 P.M.	7:00 P.M. TRF to another hosp.
F. Frank		7:30 P.M.
G. Grant	7:50 P.M.	11:39 P.M. Expired
H. Hughes	8:19 P.M.	
I. Ingals		9:15 P.M.
J. Jones	11:45 P.M.	

Calculate:

a. IP census at midnight on June 1.

b. DIPC at midnight on June 1.

c. Census at midnight on June 1.

d. IPSD total at midnight on June 1.

C H A P T E R

4

Percentage of Occupancy

CHAPTER OUTLINE

A. Bed/Bassinet Count Terms
   1. Inpatient Bed Count or Compliment
   2. Newborn Bassinet Count
B. Rate Formula
C. Beds
   1. Unit vs. Total
   2. Excluded Beds
   3. Disaster Beds
D. Bed/Bassinet Count Day Terms
   1. Inpatient Bed Count Day
   2. Inpatient Bassinet Count Day
   3. Inpatient Bed Count Days (Total)

E. Occupancy Ratio/Percentage
   1. Adults and Children (A&C)
   2. Newborn (NB)
F. Occupancy Percentage for a Period
   1. Bed
   2. Newborn (NB)
   3. Clinical Unit
G. Change in Bed Count During a Period
H. Summary
I. Chapter 4 Test

LEARNING OBJECTIVES

After studying this chapter the learner should be able to:

1. Define "bed count" and "bed compliment."
2. Define "bassinet count."
3. Explain the "rate formula."
4. Identify the beds included and excluded in a bed count.

5. Compute bed occupancy percentage (A&C percentage).
6. Compute bassinet occupancy percentage (NB).
7. Compute occupancy percentage when there is a change in bed/bassinet count.

The census data in the previous chapter provided information about the number of patients receiving hospital service or the average number for a specified period. The percentage of occupancy provides a hospital with a ratio or percentage of the equipped and staffed hospital beds/bassinets that are occupied for a specified period of time. As previously mentioned a hospital is equipped and staffed for a designated number of beds and/or bassinets and statistical analysis is carried out to assess their utilization in terms of adult and children (A&C) occupancy or newborn (NB) occupancy.

A. BED/BASSINET COUNT TERMS

1. *Inpatient Bed Count or Bed Complement*

The number of available hospital inpatient beds, both occupied and vacant, on any given day.

2. *Newborn Bassinet Count*

The number of available hospital newborn bassinets, both occupied and vacant, on a given day.

Explanation: Hospitals are generally licensed for a certain number of beds. Hospital staffing (nursing staff, housekeeping staff, laboratory personnel, etc.) is based on the beds available and therefore it would *not* be cost effective to staff empty beds.

Adding/Decreasing: Hospitals often open and close nursing units based on need. During periods of diminished demand, a clinical nursing unit may be closed, and, during periods of peak demand, another unit may be opened. The opening of an additional unit will add to the bed count, whereas the closing of a clinical nursing unit will decrease the bed count (available beds). As units are opened or closed, the staffing needs for the hospital change as well.

Example: A medical unit may close in December and be reopened in January if a need exists. Many hospital administrative decisions are based on hospital occupancy percentages. Therefore, it is important that the occupancy figures be accurate. A hospital does not want to be overstaffed and lose money, nor does a community want to have an inadequate number of beds to meet the medical needs of its constituency, if such a situation can be avoided.

B. RATE FORMULA

All of the rates that follow can be determined by keeping in mind a general rule that applies to computing rates. A rate is:

$$\frac{\text{The number of times something happens}}{\text{The number of times it } could \text{ happen}}$$

Example: A person is shooting baskets and takes 25 shots at the basket. The ball goes through the basketball hoop 15 times. It can then be said the individual scored 15/25 times or successfully completed 60% of the shots.

Hospital Example: A hospital offers an AIDS blood test to every hospital employee and 200 employees sign up for the test. The hospital has a total of 400 employees. Therefore,

200/400 employees signed up for the AIDS test, or it could be said that 50% of the employees will be tested.

School Example: There are 50 questions on a scheduled exam. You answer 40 questions correctly. Your score on the exam is 40/50 or 80% of the questions were answered correctly.

C. BEDS

1. Unit vs. Totals

Again, as mentioned earlier, the use of the singular form of the word "day" in a title indicates a unit of measure. The inpatient bed count day is a unit of measure indicating the number of beds that are set up, staffed, and equipped for patient care on a particular day.

The use of the word "days" is a total and indicates the total for the days in a period—week, month, three months, year, etc.

2. Excluded Beds

There are some beds in a hospital that are available in other than patient rooms. One of these beds is occupied by a patient primarily on a temporary basis while the patient is examined or treated in another area of the hospital. The patient has been assigned a hospital bed on a clinical nursing unit but leaves that bed or area for treatment or examination elsewhere. These excluded beds include beds in examining rooms, physical therapy beds, labor room beds, recovery room beds (following surgery), and beds in the ER. Normally, ER beds are occupied by outpatients during the time of treatment, after which the outpatient is released from the hospital. However, some patients are admitted after being seen in the ER. However, these patients were not inpatients at the time of the ER visit and are assigned a hospital bed and room on admission.

Example: A patient is admitted to room 205 (surgical unit) on December 3. On December 4 the patient is taken to surgery. Following surgery, the patient is taken to the recovery room before being returned to his/her assigned room of 205. The patient is considered to be a patient in 205 throughout this time even though the patient will have occupied a temporary bed in the operating room and recovery room. If, however, the patient is taken to ICU following surgery, the patient is TRF-out of 205 and TRF-in to ICU on December 4, as previously mentioned in Chapter 3 regarding census data.

3. Disaster Beds

Occasionally, at the time of a disaster (earthquake, train derailment, tornado, nuclear disaster, etc.) or during periods of epidemics (such as flu epidemics), all the regular hospital beds are occupied. Most hospitals have extra beds that may be available for set-up during these peak periods. In some instances these beds are set up in lounges, hallways, and other rooms that are not normally patient rooms. These extra beds *do not* become a part of the inpatient bed count, but the patients occupying the beds are counted in the census and census statistics that include inpatient service days.

D. BED/BASSINET COUNT DAY TERMS

A "bed count day" shares similarities with the concept of an inpatient service day, since it is thought of as one patient occupying one bed for a specified day/days. The term *bed count* applies to all the beds available for inpatient use that are set up and staffed.

1. ***Inpatient Bed Count Day***

   A unit of measure denoting the presence of one inpatient bed, set up and staffed for use and either occupied or vacant, during one 24-hour period.

2. ***Inpatient Bassinet Count Day***

   A unit of measure denoting the presence of one inpatient bassinet, set up and staffed for use and either occupied or vacant, during one 24-hour period.

3. ***Inpatient Bed Count Days (Total)***

   The sum of inpatient bed count days during the period under consideration.

E. OCCUPANCY RATIO/PERCENTAGE

Occupancy percentages (also called rates or ratios) state the percentage of the available beds or bassinets that are being utilized (occupied) on a specific day or for a designated period of time—that is, the percentage of use or utilization.

1. ***Adults and Children (A&C)***

   a. *Inpatient Bed Occupancy Ratio*

      The proportion of inpatient beds occupied, defined as the ratio of service days to inpatient bed count days in the period under consideration.

   b. *Formula: Daily Inpatient Bed Occupancy Percentage*

   $$\frac{\text{Daily IP census (IP service days)}}{\text{Inpatient bed count for that day}} \times 100$$

   c. *Explanation*

      Relating the formula for computing rates to computing bed occupancy ratio or percentage involves finding what percentage of beds are filled on a given date or for a period of time. As mentioned, the bed count has been established at the beginning of a period and is the number of beds available that are set up and staffed.

   d. *All Beds Occupied*

      1) *One Day*

         If every hospital bed is occupied on a specific day, the bed occupancy percentage for that day would be 100%.

      2) *Period*

         If every hospital bed is occupied during a certain period of time (say, one week) the bed occupancy percentage for that (one-week) period would be 100%. However, this is not generally the case nor would it constitute good management, because hospitals would plan to have a few beds available for emergency situations. Hospitals plan to have occupancy rates of 90%, but this is often not achieved, especially during the last few years as fewer patients have been treated on an inpatient basis and more and more patients have been treated as outpatients. Also, shorter stays are more commonly the rule, especially for Medicare patients, although certainly all insurance companies are trying to cut costs wherever possible. This trend has mandated greater utilization of outpatient treatment and shorter inpatient stays.

e. **Disaster Beds and Occupancy Rates**

Occasionally disasters occur and every bed count bed is occupied. At such times additional beds are added, as already mentioned. When this occurs the bed count does *not* change, because these disaster beds are *not* included in the established bed count. However, the patient is counted, and therefore the bed occupancy percentage could be greater than 100%.

Example: A hospital is a 200-bed hospital (200 beds being routinely set up and staffed daily). A tornado hits the area and all 200 beds are assigned and occupied. Five additional beds are set up and patients are admitted to these beds. The percentage of bed occupancy on that day would be 205/200—the number of inpatients present (205) divided by the bed count (200). This is an example of a circumstance that would result in a bed occupancy percentage of greater than 100%.

f. **Normal Occupancy Percentage**

In most cases, a hospital's bed occupancy percentage is less than 100%. In the general day-to-day operation of a hospital not all beds are occupied. A 200-bed hospital that has 180 patients on a specific day has a bed occupancy percentage of 180/200, or 90%. If on the following day the inpatient service day total is 175, the bed occupancy percentage falls to 175/200, or 87.5%. In this manner, the percentage of bed occupancy can be determined each day.

2. **Newborn (NB)**

a. **Formula: Daily Newborn Bassinet Occupancy Percentage**

$$\frac{\text{Daily NB census (IP service days)}}{\text{NB bassinet count for that day}} \times 100$$

b. **Example**

A NB nursery has 10 bassinets. On a specific day the daily NB census is 8 newborns. The daily newborn bassinet count for that day is 8/10, or 80%, occupancy.

SELF-TEST 19

Compute the answers correctly to *one* decimal place.

1. A 300-bed hospital has 185 of its beds occupied on February 20. What is the percentage of bed occupancy for February 20?

2. On May 5, a hospital with 85 beds has an inpatient service day total of 60 patients. What is the percentage of bed occupancy for May 5?

3. On September 10, an explosion occurs in a chemical plant and a daily inpatient census of 160 patients was recorded by the local 150-bed hospital. What is the bed occupancy percentage for September 10?

4. On January 8, the midnight census is 120. However, five patients were admitted and discharged that same day. The hospital has a bed complement of 130 beds. What is the bed occupancy percentage for January 8?

5. On March 6, a total of 12 bassinets are occupied out of a bassinet count of 15. On March 7 three babies are born live and one is stillborn. That same day two babies are discharged home with their mothers. What is the bassinet occupancy percentage for March 7?

6. The following statistics are recorded on the Neonatal Unit on June 8:

Bassinet count	12
Beginning census (midnight on June 7)	9
Births	3
NB discharges (live)	4
NB death	1
Fetal death	1

    Calculate:

    a. Inpatient service day total for the unit on June 8.

    b. Bassinet occupancy percentage for the unit on June 8.

F. OCCUPANCY PERCENTAGE FOR A PERIOD

Generally, for long-term planning it is necessary to know the percentage of occupancy over a longer period of time than just a day. Individual day rates can vary greatly and it is more helpful to see the percentage for a period (a month, for instance) than to study the individual percentages for each day in that period (in this case, a month).

1. Bed

Formula: Inpatient Bed Occupancy Percentage for a Period

$$\frac{\text{Total inpatient service days for a period}}{\text{Total IP bed count days} \times \text{number of days in period}} \times 100$$

Example: Suppose Pleasantville Hospital is a 50-bed hospital. In June a total of 1410 inpatient service days were documented. To calculate the percentage of bed occupancy for the month of June, the total of 1410 IP service days is placed in the numerator and this is divided by 50×30 (or 1500) and the final result multiplied by 100 to convert it to a percentage, or 94%.

Example: In June, 1200 inpatients were serviced in a 50-bed hospital. The numerator in this example is 1200 (IP service days) and the denominator is 50×30 (since there are 30 days in June). Thus 1200 divided by 1500 is 0.80, which is multiplied by 100, giving 80%.

Note: Always be sure to use IP service days for the numerator rather than census-taking time data.

2. Newborn (NB)

Formula: Newborn Bassinet Occupancy Percentage for a Period

$$\frac{\text{Total NB IP service days for a period}}{\text{Total NB bassinet count} \times \text{number of days in period}} \times 100$$

Example: Caring Hospital has a bassinet count of 30. During July, a total of 825 NB inpatient service days of care were given. To calculate the percentage of occupancy for the newborn bassinets, the total of 825 is divided by the product of 30×31 (or 930) and the result multiplied by 100 to convert it into a percentage. This results in a percentage of 88.7% $[(825 \div 930) \times 100]$.

3. Clinical Unit

Formula: Clinical Unit Occupancy Percentage for a Period

$$\frac{\text{Total IP service days for a clinical unit for a period}}{\text{IP bed count total for that unit} \times \text{number of days in the period}} \times 100$$

Example: The pediatric unit of a hospital has 15 beds. During the first week of October, the IP service day totals were 12, 11, 13, 9, 10, 13, 7. To find the occupancy percentage for the week, first total the IP service days $(12 + 11 + 13 + 9 + 10 + 13 + 7)$, which equals 75. Then divide by the product of the bed count (15) $\times$ number of days (7), which yields 105. Finally, multiply the quotient by 100 to convert it to a percent. The result is 71.4% $[(75 \div 105) \times 100]$.

SELF-TEST 20

Carry answers correctly to *two* decimal places.
1. A clinical unit with a bed count of 18 beds reports the following figures for December:

	IP Service Days
Dec. 1 through Dec. 10	165
Dec. 11 through Dec. 20	162
Dec. 21 through Dec. 31	180

Calculate:

a. Period with the best bed occupancy percentage.

b. Inpatient bed occupancy percentage for the month of December.

2. St. Teresa Hospital records the following data:

	IP Service Days	Bed Count
January through April	18,850	175
May through July	17,340	200
August through October	13,220	150
November through December	8,880	165

Calculate: Period with the best inpatient bed occupancy percentage.

3. The daily inpatient service day totals for a 50-bed hospital are as follows:

Feb.	1	40	Feb.	8	37	Feb.	15	38	Feb.	22	41
	2	41		9	48		16	48		23	45
	3	43		10	46		17	44		24	46
	4	50		11	43		18	49		25	37
	5	47		12	49		19	50		26	39
	6	46		13	39		20	47		27	43
	7	38		14	48		21	40		28	48

Calculate:

a. Inpatient occupancy percentage for February 14.

b. Day with the highest inpatient occupancy percentage in February, without figuring the individual percentages.

c. Inpatient bed occupancy percentage for February.

d. Dividing the month into four equal periods of seven days each, indicate the period with the highest inpatient bed occupancy percentage—Feb. 1 through 7; Feb. 8 through 14; Feb. 15 through 21; or Feb. 22 through 28—and the bed occupancy percentage for each period.

4. A newborn unit records the following data for April:

Bassinet count	14
IP service day total	388
Beginning census	12
Admissions	88
Discharges	88
Newborn deaths	1
Fetal deaths	3

Calculate:

a. Bassinet occupancy percentage for April.

b. *(R3) Census at the end of April.

5. November data for St. John Hospital:

Clinical Unit	*IP Service Days*	*Bed/Bassinet Count*
Medical	2850	100
Surgical	988	34
Pediatric	422	15
Orthopedic	502	18
Obstetric	544	20
Newborn	524	18

Calculate:

a. Bed/bassinet occupancy percentage for each clinical unit and the unit with the best inpatient occupancy percentage for the month of November.

b. A&C inpatient bed occupancy percentage for November for St. John Hospital.

G. CHANGE IN BED COUNT DURING A PERIOD

Occasionally a hospital changes its official bed or bassinet count during a period. A hospital may expand or decrease the number of available beds. This expansion or decrease is *not* a temporary change due to an emergency, as mentioned under disaster beds, but rather a fairly permanent change for a specified period of time. Sometimes a wing of a hospital is added (increasing the bed count) or a previous wing is converted to another function (office space or laboratory space, for example) and the beds in the wing would no longer be available for patient care.

Formula: Occupancy Percentage with a Change in Bed Count During a Period

$$\frac{\text{Total IP service days for the period}}{(\text{Bed count} \times \text{days}) + (\text{Bed count} \times \text{days})} \times 100$$

(Days refers to the number of days in the period.)

Example: Jubilee Hospital has decided to expand its facilities and add additional beds. The January through June bed count was 200 beds. On July 1, an additional 20 beds were added. The total number of inpatient service days for the first six-month period was 36,006 and for the second six-month period the total was 40,004. To compute the inpatient bed occupancy percentage, add the IP service days for the year (36,006 + 40,004 = 76,010) and divide by the sum of the two (bed count times days) periods (200 beds × 181 days) + (220 beds × 184 days) or 36,200 + 40,480 = 76,680. Carrying out the division (76,010 divided by 76,680), and then multiplying by 100, results in an inpatient bed occupancy percentage of 99.1%.

Example: Sunshine Hospital begins the year with an official bed count of 50 beds. On January 15, another 10 beds are officially added, for a bed count total of 60 beds. The inpatient service day total for January was 1680. To find the inpatient bed occupancy percentage for January, divide the IP service day total (1680) by the denominator [(50 × 14) + (60 × 17) = 700 + 1020 = 1720] or (1680 divided by 1720). Multiplying the result by 100 gives a 97.67% inpatient occupancy percentage for January.

SELF-TEST 21

Answers should be correct to *two* decimal places.

1. Expansion Hospital begins the year with a total of 150 beds and 10 bassinets.

   On March 1, 15 additional beds are added to the bed count, for a total of 165 beds.

   On April 1, an additional 5 bassinets are added to the newborn nursery, for a total of 15 bassinets.

   On July 1, the hospital expands again, this time adding another 15 beds and 5 bassinets, bringing the total counts to 180 beds and 20 bassinets.

On October 1, another expansion occurs and 20 additional beds are added, for a total bed complement of 200 beds. The service day totals for the periods are as follows:

Period	IP Service Days		Counts	
	Bed	*Bassinet*	*Bed*	*Bassinet*
Jan. through Feb.	8550	555	150	10
Mar.	4775	288	165	10
Apr. through June	14,425	1242	165	15
July through Sept.	16,005	1666	180	20
Oct. through Dec.	17,704	1744	200	20

Calculate:

a. IP bed occupancy percentage for each quarter (Jan. through Mar.; Apr. through June; July through Sept.; Oct. through Dec.).

b. Newborn occupancy percentage for each quarter.

c. IP bed occupancy percentage for the year.

d. Newborn bassinet occupancy percentage for the year.

e. Quarter with the best IP bed occupancy percentage.

2. Prairie Hospital, with a complement of 250 beds, finds it difficult to make ends meet due to low occupancy. The administration decides to close a wing of the hospital and the administrative closure is implemented on July 17, reducing the bed count to 200 beds. During July, 5710 IP service days of care were given.

   Calculate: Percent of IP bed occupancy for July.

3. A total of 76,006 IP service days of care were given at Blessing Hospital during a non-leap year. The bed counts changed from a count of 200 at the beginning of the year to 220 on March 15, and then to 230 on July 1. The count was reduced to 210 on November 15 and it remained at that level through the end of the year.

   Calculate: IP bed occupancy percentage for the year.

4. The newborn nursery rendered a total of 676 patient days of care during January. The bassinet count was 25 on January 1 but changed to 18 on January 22.

   Calculate: Bassinet occupancy percentage for January.

5. General Hospital reported the following for a non-leap year:

Period	IPSD		Count	
	A&C	*NB*	*Bed*	*Bassinet*
Jan. 1 through Jan. 31	4880	601	160	20
Feb. through March	10,115	1110	180	20
Apr. through June	16,662	2190	200	25
July through Sept.	15,558	2069	175	25
Oct. through Dec.	15,612	1722	175	20

Calculate:

a. IP bed occupancy percentage for January.

b. Bassinet occupancy percentage for February through March.

c. IP bed occupancy for the first half of the year (January through June).

d. Bassinet occupancy percentage for the second half of the year (July through December).

e. IP bed occupancy percentage for the entire year.

f. Bassinet occupancy percentage for the entire year.

g. Quarter with the best IP bed occupancy percentage during the year.

h. Quarter with the best bassinet occupancy percentage for the year.

6. On January 11, a 50-bed hospital added 10 beds, for a total of 60 beds. On January 21, another 10 beds were added, for a total of 70 beds. The inpatient service days for the period were 1800.

Calculate:

a. Inpatient bed occupancy percentage for January.

b. If the hospital reduced the beds from 70 to 60 on February 1 and maintained that bed count through February, with a February IP service day total of 1250, what is the inpatient bed occupancy percentage for the entire period (January through February) if the year is a non-leap year?

H. SUMMARY

1. Bed count/bed complement includes beds set up and staffed, either vacant or occupied.
2. Bassinet count includes bassinets set up and staffed, either vacant or occupied.
3. Bed occupancy includes all adults and children admitted to the hospital. Beds are also assigned to newborns and infants not born in the hospital during that particular

admission, such as babies born en route or admitted after being born and infants only hours or days old.

4. Bassinet occupancy includes only newborns born in the hospital during that admission and admitted to the neonatal unit.
5. Excluded beds from a bed count:
   a. Examining room beds—ER beds
   b. Treatment room beds—labor beds

          —recovery room beds

          —ER room beds

          —observation beds

          —23 hours hold

          —physical therapy beds

          —outpatient surgery beds
6. Disaster beds. These beds are added during emergency situations (during a time of disaster), are temporary, and are *not* included in a bed count.
7. Rate. A rate is the number of times something happens divided by the number of times it could have happened.
8. Percentage of occupancy.
   a. Separate percentages are figured for A&C and NB. These are generally *not* combined.
   b. Be sure to use IPSD in the numerator.
   c. Daily percentage.
      Divide the IPSD by the bed/bassinet count.
   d. Period percentage.
      Divide the IPSD by the bed/bassinet count × number of days in the period.
   e. Change in bed count percentage.
      Divide the IPSD by the bed/bassinet count × number of days in the period + (beds × days) + (beds × days)—one for each period with a different bed count.
   f. Disaster beds. If all beds are occupied and temporary beds are set up (as in a disaster), the percentage of occupancy will be greater than 100%.
   g. Clinical unit percentages are computed in the same manner as the bed/bassinet counts.

I. CHAPTER 4 TEST

Note: Compute all answers correctly to *two* decimal places.

1. Recorded for May for a 65-bed hospital:

		IPSD			IPSD			IPSD
May	1	50	May	11	48	May	21	55
	2	50		12	56		22	58
	3	49		13	58		23	62
	4	54		14	56		24	65
	5	52		15	59		25	63
	6	51		16	60		26	62
	7	50		17	59		27	60
	8	43		18	58		28	60
	9	44		19	54		29	62
	10	46		20	55		30	63
							31	50

Calculate:

a. Percentage of occupancy for the month of May.

b. Percentage of occupancy for May 25.

c. Percentage of occupancy for:

   1) May 1 through May 10.

   2) May 11 through May 20.

   3) May 21 through May 31.

d. Percentage of occupancy for May if the bed count had increased to 70 beds on May 11 and to 75 beds on May 21.

2. Blessing Hospital

		A&C	NB	Surgical
Bed/bassinet count		100	10	25
Feb. 9:	Census	95	8	18
Feb. 10:	Admissions	8	2	4
	Disch. (live)	5	1	2
	Deaths	1	0	1
	A&D	2	0	0

Calculate:

a. A&C bed occupancy percentage for February 10.

b. NB bassinet occupancy percentage for February 10.

c. Surgical Unit bed occupancy percentage for February 10.

d. *(R3) Census for February 10.

3. High Hopes Hospital (Neonatal Unit: 16 bassinets)

Jan. 1:	Census	13
Jan. 2:	Births	4
	Disch. (live)	2
	Deaths (NB)	1
	Deaths (fetal)	1 (late fetal)
	A&D	1

Calculate:

a. *(R3) Census for January 2.

b. *(R3) IPSD total for January 2.

c. Bassinet occupancy percentage for January 2.

4. St. Vincent Hospital

	Bed		Bassinet		Surgical	
Period	**Count**	**IPSD**	**Count**	**IPSD**	**Count**	**IPSD**
Jan. through Mar.	160	12,405	18	1,378	25	2,180
Apr. through June	180	14,621	15	1,247	30	2,516
July through Sept.	200	15,777	20	1,615	30	2,601
Oct. through Dec.	175	14,813	25	2,084	35	2,913

Calculate:

a. Percentage of occupancy for each period for the following:

   1) Bed percentage

   2) Bassinet percentage

   3) Surgical unit percentage

b. Category (bed, bassinet, or surgical unit) with the best percentage of occupancy for the year.

5.   Golden Valley Hospital

		A&C	NB	Orthopedic
Bed/bassinet count		80	10	12
Beginning census		74	7	6
March:	Admissions	105	57	47
	Disch. (live)	99	54	44
	Deaths	5	1	2
	A&D	45	3	4
	IPSD	1998	268	278

Calculate:

a.   Bed (A&C) occupancy percentage for March.

b.   Bassinet (NB) occupancy percentage for March.

c.   Orthopedic unit occupancy percentage for March.

6.   Comforting Hospital (for November)

	Count		
Units:	**Bed**	**Bassinet**	**IPSD**
Medical	58		1660
Surgical	32		886
Pediatrics	10		215
Orthopedics	18		498
Ophthalmology	25		702
Obstetrics	15		405
Newborn	____	12	324
Totals	158	12	

Calculate:

a.   Percentage of occupancy for each unit for November.

b.   A&C percentage of occupancy for November.

c.   Percentage of occupancy for the entire hospital.

7. Hilltop Hospital

| Period | Dates | Counts | | IPSD | |
		Beds	Bassinets	Beds	Bassinets
A	Jan. 1 through Feb. 15	90	12	3815	463
B	Feb. 16 through Mar. 31	100	8	4079	314
C	Apr. 1 through Apr. 30	110	10	2986	272
D	May 1 through June 30	85	14	4021	708

Calculate:

a. Percentage of bed occupancy for each period;

   Percentage of bassinet occupancy for each period.

b. Percentage of bed occupancy for January through June;

   Percentage of bassinet occupancy for January through June.

c. Period with the best IP bed occupancy percentage.

8. Mountain View Hospital

Period	Bed Count	IPSD
Jan.	250	6250
Feb.	225	5984
Mar.	200	5888
Apr. through June	210	17,920
July through Sept.	200	17,561
Oct. through Dec.	180	16,007

Calculate:

a. Bed occupancy percentage for January.

b. Bed occupancy percentage for February through March.

c. Bed occupancy percentage for the first half of the year.

d. Bed occupancy percentage for the second half of the year.

e. Bed occupancy percentage for the entire year.

f. Quarter with the best bed occupancy percentage for the year.

9.   Holy Cross Hospital
     Bed count: 50

		IPSD			**IPSD**			**IPSD**
June	1	45	June	11	35	June	21	44
	2	30		12	41		22	48
	3	35		13	47		23	35
	4	25		14	48		24	36
	5	47		15	49		25	38
	6	48		16	50		26	42
	7	38		17	40		27	44
	8	42		18	41		28	40
	9	43		19	43		29	52
	10	36		20	47		30	41

Calculate:

a.   *(R3) Total IPSD for June.

b.   *(R3) IPSD for June 7 through June 15.

c.   *(R3) Average DIPC for June 1 through June 10.

d.   *(R3) Average IPSD for June.

e.   Percentage of bed occupancy for June.

f.   Percentage of bed occupancy for June 29.

g.   If the bed count had increased to 55 beds on June 15, calculate the percentage of occupancy for June.

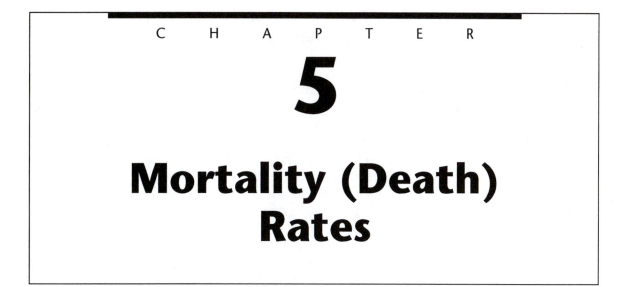

CHAPTER

5

Mortality (Death) Rates

CHAPTER OUTLINE

A. Terms
  1. Mortality
  2. Morbidity
  3. Discharge
  4. Death
  5. Net vs. Gross
B. Death Rates
  1. Gross Death Rate
  2. Net Death Rate or Institutional Death Rate

  3. Helpful Hints
  4. Newborn Death Rate
  5. Surgical Death Rates
  6. Maternal Death Rate
  7. Fetal Death Rate
C. Summary
D. Chapter 5 Test

LEARNING OBJECTIVES

After studying this chapter the learner should be able to:

1. Distinguish clearly between
   a. Mortality vs. Morbidity
   b. Net vs. Gross
2. Describe what is included in a "discharge."
3. Identify deaths that are excluded in gross and net death rates.

4. Compute the following death rates:
   a. Gross
   b. Net
   c. Newborn (Infant)
   d. Postoperative
   e. Anesthesia
   f. Maternal
   g. Fetal (Stillborn)

Up to now all calculations have been carried out on *admission data*, by counting each patient who has received service on a specified day and totaling the daily total for various specified periods. Also, the inpatient bed and bassinet occupancy percentages were also calculated on the basis of how many patients were present in the hospital each day.

The majority of the remaining statistical computations will be based on *discharge data* accumulated at the time of discharge. In other words, all the services a patient may need during his/her hospitalization cannot be ascertained precisely at the time of admission. However, once a patient leaves the hospital (upon discharge), this additional information is obtainable and evaluations can be made not only about services received (quantity) but also about the effectiveness or quality of that care.

A discharge occurs at the end of a patient's hospitalization. A discharge order should be written on a patient when the physician determines that the patient may be released from the facility. The absence of a discharge order may indicate that the patient left the hospital against medical advice (AMA), though the patient will be included in the discharge statistics. Another type of discharge is a death, so the term *discharge* includes those discharged either dead or alive. If the term *live discharges* is used, the deaths need to be added in to arrive at the total discharges for that date or period of time.

Inpatient deaths are those that occur during a patient's inpatient hospitalization and are included in the hospital's mortality (death) rate. Outpatient deaths are those that occur at a time other than during hospitalization as an inpatient. The patient who dies at home or en route to the hospital or during an outpatient procedure is an outpatient death.

A major change to keep in mind regarding statistical treatment is that, in computing death rates, newborns are combined with adults and children, instead of determining each category separately, as was done with census data (based on admission data). Unless the death rate specifies a specific group (such as a newborn death rate), all inpatient deaths should be included when computing death rates.

A. TERMS:

1. *Mortality*

Mortality refers to death or being fatal—a fatality. A mortal is subject to death or is destined to die. Mortality rates are death rates.

2. *Morbidity*

Do not confuse mortality with morbidity. Morbidity refers to being diseased. A morbid condition pertains to disease or being affected by disease. Morbidity refers to the sick rate or the ratio of sick to well.

3. *Discharge*

Each patient admitted to the hospital sooner or later leaves the hospital and is considered discharged. Remember that the term *discharge* includes a patient who is discharged home, discharged to an extended care facility (nursing home, rehabilitation facility, etc.), transfers to another hospital, or expires in the hospital. A death is considered a discharge.

4. *Death*

a. *Inpatient Death*

A death is included in the term discharge and describes a patient who expires while a patient in the hospital. Remember that our primary concern here is inpatient statistical treatment. Therefore, an inpatient death applies to a patient who expires after admission to the hospital as an inpatient (as opposed to an outpatient death).

b. **Non-Inpatient Death**

The following deaths are *not* to be included when computing IP death rates:

1) *Emergency Room (ER) Death*

A patient who is seen in the emergency room and dies prior to admission to an inpatient bed is considered an outpatient death.

2) *Dead on Arrival (DOA)*

A patient who is DOA at the hospital also was never an inpatient. In the majority of cases, an attempt at resuscitating the patient is made in the emergency room, but the patient was never an inpatient admission so would *not* be an inpatient death.

3) *Outpatient (OP) Death*

Some patients are administered treatment in a hospital as an outpatient. These patients may be at your facility for outpatient surgery or for an exercise EKG to assess their cardiac status or for a nuclear medicine scan, to name just a few of the reasons for outpatient treatment or assessment. Some patients are also admitted to home care, are on a specified regimen, and are followed up by their physician, home care nurses, or health care professional. Again, these patients do *not* fit the criteria for an inpatient death but, should they die, they are categorized as outpatient deaths.

4) *Hospital Fetal Death (Abortion/Stillborn Infant)*

The term fetal death is preferred over the more common term of "stillbirth" or "aborted fetus." A hospital fetal death is death *prior* to the complete expulsion or extraction from its mother, in a hospital facility, of a product of human conception, fetus and placenta, irrespective of the duration of pregnancy. The death is indicated by the fact that after such expulsion or extraction, the fetus does not breathe or show any other evidence of life, such as beating of the heart, pulsation of the umbilical cord, or definite movement of voluntary muscles.

Again, because such a fetus was born dead and did not show any signs of life, a fetal death would *never* be included as an inpatient or used in determining IP death rates. Furthermore, a fetal death is not categorized as an OP death. However, even though data are kept on the number of fetal deaths, the number is *only* used in figuring fetal death rates.

Designations of fetal death by *gestational* age:

Early—Less than 20 weeks gestation.
Intermediate—20 weeks to less than 28 weeks.
Late—28 or more weeks gestation.

Designations of fetal death by *gram weight*:

Early—500 grams or less.
Intermediate—501 to 1000 grams.
Late—1001 grams or more.

Comparisons of grams to pounds:

1000 grams = 2 lb 3 oz
2500 grams = 5 lb 8 oz

Premature birth applies to a newborn with a birth weight of less than 2500 grams.

c. *Newborn Death*

It is imperative that a fetal death not be confused with a newborn death. A newborn death occurs in an infant who was born *alive* and dies *after* birth. A fetal death showed no signs of life at the time of birth. Any sign of life indicates a *live* birth, even if death occurs minutes after birth. In this instance, the death would be classified as a newborn death rather than a fetal death.

5. Net vs. Gross

Whenever the term *gross* is used statistically, it represents an amount before anything is subtracted or, in the case of death rates, it includes all deaths (inpatient here) with no exclusions. This is analogous to working pay. An employee, for instance, is hired to work a forty-hour work week at a pay rate of five dollars an hour. This employee will have an earned gross pay of $200.00 a week (hourly rate × hours worked, or $5.00 × 40 hours). However, seldom does a worker take home the *gross* amount because the employer generally deducts something from that gross pay before the employee receives the paycheck. (These deductions may include federal and state income tax, social security, retirement fund, hospital insurance, etc.) The amount that the employee takes home (amount on the paycheck) is the employee's *net* pay. The *net* pay is the gross pay minus the deductions. It is important to keep in mind that whenever the term *net rate* is used, something will need to be subtracted. *Gross − something = net.*

B. DEATH RATES

Based on discharge data, a list is prepared of all patients who died during their hospital stay. From these lists or counts the death rate can be determined. Remember that, upon discharge, a patient is classified as being discharged either alive or dead and that the term discharge includes death. However, look at the data carefully, because the term *live discharges* is also used, in which case the live discharges must be added to the deaths to determine the total discharges.

Example: On January 15, fifteen patients were discharged. Of these 15, two were deaths and 13 were live discharges.

Hint: Keep in mind the formula for determining any rate—divide the number of times something happens by the number of times it *could* happen. When in doubt about what data to use in a formula, recall this reminder.

1. Gross Death Rate

Formula:

$$\frac{\text{Total number of deaths (including NB) for a period}}{\text{Total number of discharges (including deaths) for the period (NB and A\&C)}} \times 100$$

Example: If 100 patients are discharged in a certain month and three of these were deaths, the result is a gross death rate of 3% (3 ÷ 100 = 0.03, which is multiplied by 100).

Explanation: When confused, recall the general rate formula. As you reason out the answer, it becomes clear that any patient who is hospitalized may die during hospitalization. In the example above, three patients expired. However, remember to use *discharge data*, since any patient who is still hospitalized could die before discharge and only upon discharge would it be known whether the patient survived or died. Therefore, death rates are not figured on currently hospitalized patients (census data) but rather on patients who have been discharged (discharge data).

2. *Net Death Rate or Institutional Death Rate*

Formula:

$$\frac{\text{Total IP deaths (incl. NB) minus those under 48 hours for a period}}{\text{Total discharges minus deaths under 48 hours for the period}} \times 100$$

(Remember that discharges include deaths and that NBs—deaths and discharges—are included in the denominator as well.)

Explanation: The thinking behind this formula includes the belief that if a patient expires in less than 48 hours there was insufficient time to diagnose and treat a life-threatening disorder and that only emergency and stabilizing treatment could be provided during such a short period of time. For this reason, the institutional death rate came into use. To adequately assess deaths based on a more sufficient treatment time frame, the net death rate is often used. It is felt that the net death rate reflects more accurately the hospital's ability to save lives.

Hospital deaths are reviewed by a medical staff committee to determine whether appropriate care was administered and to evaluate whether other measures may have helped to save the patient's life, in hopes that lives might be saved in the future. This points to another role of statistical treatment of data. Not only are statistics important for administrative decisions (such as whether to close down a wing of the hospital) but for peer review and better patient care as well.

Not all hospitals will use this *net* or *institutional death rate;* and each hospital will determine whether it wants to keep these data. It is important to specify whether a death rate is a *gross* or *net* death rate. The term *net* indicates that certain deaths (deaths occurring less than 48 hours after admission) are *not* included and will be *subtracted* from the death total. Because these deaths are excluded in the numerator, they must also be excluded (subtracted) in the denominator (since they were neither a live discharge nor a death that occurred more than 48 hours after admission).

Example: A total of five patients expired in June, of which two died less than 48 hours and three died more than 48 hours after admission. A total of 450 inpatients were discharged in June.

Gross death rate is total deaths over total discharges (5 divided by 450), then multiplied by 100, which gives a gross death rate of 1.11%.

Net death rate only includes patients who died at least 48 hours after admission, or 3 divided by 450 minus 2 (3 ÷ 448), multiplied by 100, which gives a net death rate of 0.67%.

3. Helpful Hints

a. *Death rates should be low.* In previous calculations, high percentages based on census/inpatient service data were the norm, with high percentages being advantageous and expected. The opposite should hold true for death rates. A result of 90% (or even 20%) would clearly indicate a miscalculation and that errors should be sought. In many instances, the death rate will be less than 1%, resulting in a decimal figure (for example, 0.67% or 0.95%). Carefully check the placement of the decimal point. If an actual death rate was 0.95%, a misplaced decimal point could result in an incorrect death rate of 9.5% or, even worse, 95%.

b. *Death rates should be carried out to three (or at least two) decimal places and corrected to two (or one) places.* A tenth of a percent of a large number is less significant than a tenth of a percent of a small number. Since death rates will typically be low, calculations should be carried out further than the other calculations that have been introduced up to this point.

c. *Most death rates use* discharge *data,* not admission data. Remember: As long as a patient is hospitalized there is a chance that the patient may die and therefore discharge figures are used to calculate death rates. Any exception to this rule will be noted in the appropriate death rate.

d. *Most death rates combine NB and adults and children data.* Death rates can be figured separately (NB separately and A&C separately), but in the majority of cases they are combined. This is in contrast to census data and occupancy percentages.

4. Newborn Death Rate (Infant Death Rate or Infant Mortality Rate)

Formula:

$$\frac{\text{Total number of NB deaths for a period}}{\substack{\text{Total number of NB discharges for the period} \\ \text{(Include deaths in the discharges.)}}} \times 100$$

Example: A total of two newborns died during the month of December and there were 102 live discharges. To find the NB death rate, the two deaths are placed in the numerator and the total discharges (live and deaths), or 102 + 2 = 104, are placed in the denominator. This gives a newborn death rate of 2 divided by 104 multiplied by 100, for a percentage of 1.92% [(2 ÷ 104) × 100].

SELF-TEST 22

Compute all answers correctly to *one* decimal place.

1. Snowflake Hospital recorded the following data for May:

	Admissions	Discharges	Deaths <48 hrs	Deaths >48 hrs
Adults/Children	686	691	6	30
Newborn	58	60	1	4

Calculate:

a. Gross death rate.

b. Net death rate.

c. Infant mortality rate.

2. The following data are recorded for November:

Service	Admissions	Deaths <48 hrs	Deaths >48 hrs	Discharges
Medical	250	5	20	261
Surgical	105	2	8	103
Pediatric	33	0	2	35
Obstetrical	36	1	0	34
Psychiatric	47	1	0	45
Newborn	40	1	1	38

Calculate:

a. Gross death rate.

b. Net death rate.

c. Newborn death rate.

d. Net medical service death rate.

e. Clinical service with the lowest gross death rate.

3. A newborn nursery reports the following data for February:

Bassinet count	15	
Births (admissions)	88	
Discharges	84	
Newborn deaths	2	(1 under 48 hrs; 1 over 48 hrs)
Fetal deaths	5	(2 early; 2 intermediate; 1 late)
IP service days	398	

Calculate: Gross death rate for the newborn nursery in February.

4. Morris County Hospital reports the following for November:

	Admissions	Live Discharges	Deaths <48 hrs	Deaths >48 hrs
Adults/Children	386	388	4	12
Newborn	91	95	1	2

Calculate:

a. Gross death rate for November.

b. Net death rate for November.

c. Infant mortality rate for November.

d. Gross death rate for A&C for November.

5. A hospital newborn nursery reports a total of 234 births during the month of July. During the same month there were a total of four deaths—two newborn and two fetal deaths. One of the newborn deaths occurred under 48 hours after admission; the other occurred over 48 hours. During July a total of 238 newborns were discharged. The bassinet count for the month was 15.

Calculate: Newborn death rate for July.

6. June statistics:

```
Admissions—adults/children    650
              newborn          55
Discharges—including deaths
              adults          602
              children         45
              newborn          57
```

		<48 hrs	>48 hrs
Deaths—medical	28	4	24
surgical	3	1	2
pediatric	1	0	1
obstetric	1	1	0
newborn	2	1	1
fetal (intermediate and late)	3		

Calculate:

a. Gross death rate for June.

b. Net death rate for June.

c. Newborn death rate for June.

5. *Surgical Death Rates*

Two surgical death rates are *not* based on discharges and therefore are an exception to the rule that generally applies to figuring death rates. The two rates, which are often computed, are the following:

a. Postoperative death rate.

b. Anesthesia death rate.

a. *Postoperative Death Rate*

Formula:

$$\frac{\text{Total surgical deaths within 10 days postoperative for a period}}{\text{Total patients operated upon for the period}} \times 100$$

Explanation: Whether this death rate is of value has been questioned. It is included here because it is still used frequently by some hospitals.

Note: This formula is an exception to the rule of using discharged patients as the basis for figuring death rates. Here the comparison is made between patients who died within *ten* days after an operation and all patients who were operated on during that same period. Only patients who underwent an operation are included in this formula and the death must have occured within the postoperative days. Applying the general "rate formula," the patients to whom this *could* happen are those who were operated on. This value is used in the denominator rather than patients discharged. Patients who expire late in the postoperative period (10 days or more) are considered most likely to have died as the result of a medical condition rather than because of complications due to surgery.

Example: During the month of March, a total of three postoperative deaths were reported within 10 days postop. During March, a total of 375 patients underwent operative procedures. Applying the formula, three deaths are placed in the numerator and 375 patients (the number operated on) in the denominator. Dividing 3 by 375, and then multiplying by 100, results in a postoperative death rate of 0.8% for March.

SELF-TEST 23

Compute the rates correctly to *two* decimal places.

1. The following information is given for July:

Surgical patients admitted	185
Surgical patients operated on	187
Surgical patients discharged	183
Total deaths on surgical unit	6
Total deaths postoperatively	4
Total deaths within 10 days postop	2
Total surgical procedures performed	193
Total anesthetics administered:	188

Calculate: Postoperative death rate for July.

2. Feel Good Hospital during August reported the following surgical statistics:

   Admissions   193
   Discharges   189
   Deaths   7   (3 under 48 hours; 4 over 48 hours)
                                      (5 under 10 days; 2 over 10 days)

   Operations performed   210
   Patients operated on   188

   Calculate: Postoperative death rate for August.

b. *Anesthesia Death Rate*
   Formula:

$$\frac{\text{Total deaths caused by anesthetic agents for a period}}{\text{Total number of anesthetics administered for the period}} \times 100$$

Explanation: A death due to an anesthetic agent can only be determined by a physician. Refer to Huffman (*Medical Record Management*) for further information.

Note: Anesthesia deaths occur rarely and therefore are only computed annually.

Example: During the year, 1400 anesthetic agents were administered and it was determined that one death resulted from an anesthetic agent. The yearly anesthesia death rate would be 1 divided by 1400, then multiplied by 100, for a rate of 0.07% [(1 ÷ 1400) × 100]. Be sure to check the placement of the decimal point in anesthesia death rates.

SELF-TEST 24

Compute the answers correctly to *two* decimal places.

1. Chastity Hospital reports the following surgical data for the year:

   Admissions   1843
   Discharges   1849
   Deaths   40   (9 under 48 hrs; 31 over 48 hrs)
                                      (12 under 10 days postop; 28 over 10 days postop)
                                      (2 reported due to anesthetic agent)

   Operations performed   2010
   Patients operated on   1852
   Anesthetics administered 1854

   Calculate:

   a. Anesthetic death rate for the year.

   b. Postoperative death rate for the year.

    c. Gross surgical death rate for the year.

    d. Net surgical death rate for the year.

2. In July, Blessing Hospital reported the following surgical data:

Admissions	258	
Discharges	262	
Deaths	9	(3 under 48 hrs; 6 over 48 hrs)
		(2 under 10 days postop; 7 over 10 days postop)
		(0 due to anesthetic agent)
Anesthetics administered	298	
Surgical procedures performed	301	
Patients operated on	260	

Calculate:

    a. Anesthesia death rate for July.

    b. Postoperative death rate for July.

    c. Gross surgical death rate for July.

    d. Net surgical death rate for July.

6. *Maternal Death Rate*

Formula:

$$\frac{\text{Total maternal deaths for a period}}{\text{Total maternal (obstetrical) discharges for the period (including deaths)}} \times 100$$

a. *Terms:*

1) *Maternal Death*

The death of any woman from any cause, either while pregnant or within 42 days of termination of the pregnancy, irrespective of the duration and the site of the pregnancy.

2) *Direct Maternal Death*

A death directly related to pregnancy. An example would be eclampsia or postpartum hemorrhage. Direct maternal deaths are generally the only deaths included in a maternal death rate. An indirect maternal death is included in a net or gross death rate.

3) *Indirect Maternal Death*

A maternal death *not* directly due to obstetric causes but aggravated by the pregnant condition. An example of an indirect maternal death might be a patient with diabetes mellitus who is pregnant and who dies as the result of complications from the diabetes, which was aggravated by the pregnant condition.

4) *Puerperium*

The puerperal period is a period of 42 days following delivery and is included as part of the pregnancy period. A female who has delivered a product of conception and who dies within this period due to pregnancy is also considered a maternal or obstetrical death.

5) *Delivery*

A delivery refers to expelling a product of conception or having it removed from the body. It should be pointed out that multiple births are considered a single delivery and that a woman who gives birth to twins or triplets (multiple births) is credited with one delivery.

6) *Undelivered*

Occasionally a pregnant woman is admitted to the hospital because of complications of the pregnancy and then goes home without having delivered. At the time of discharge, the patient's condition is noted as "undelivered." A woman may also be admitted following delivery because of complications and go home undelivered.

7) *Abortion*

Abortions may be either spontaneous or induced. They most commonly occur during the first trimester of pregnancy and result in an early fetal death.

8) *Partum*

Partum means childbirth.

    a) Antepartum—the period before giving birth.
    b) Postpartum—the period after giving birth.

b. **Maternal Deaths Included:**

Hospital statistics primarily include only *direct maternal* deaths, which are deaths as the result of pregnancy. Included are:

1) Abortion death—during or following an abortion.
2) Antepartum death (death prior to delivery) caused by the pregnancy.
3) Postpartum death (death after delivery) due to pregnancy.
4) Deaths at the time of delivery due to pregnancy.

c. **Deaths Not Included:**

1) Death of a pregnant woman in a car accident.
2) Death of a pregnant woman due to suicide.
3) Death of a pregnant woman not directly related to her pregnant condition (this would be a hospital death but not a maternal death).

Note: Maternal death rates should be *low* as was the case with anesthesia deaths. Therefore, the rate is most commonly computed only on a yearly basis, rather than monthly, and should be carried out to three decimal places.

If all the maternal deaths are the result of abortions, it is a good idea to attach a note to the death rate stating this fact, to avoid confusing deaths resulting from abortions with deaths in the delivery room.

Example: The year-end report from the obstetrical unit lists the following figures:

Admissions	1550
Discharges	1554
Deliveries	1488
Abortions	46
Undelivered	38
Deaths	3 (2 due to abortions; 1 following C-section)

Applying the formula, 3 deaths makes up the numerator and 1554 discharges are included in the denominator. Dividing 3 by 1554, and then multiplying by 100, results in a maternal death rate of 0.19% for the year.

SELF-TEST 25

Compute the answers correctly to *two* decimal places.

1. The obstetrical unit reported five deaths of pregnant females for the year. The causes of death are listed as follows:

    Puerperal septicemia
    Toxemia of pregnancy
    Ruptured ectopic (tubal) pregnancy
    Leukemia aggravated by pregnancy
    Placental hemorrhaging due to a fall down the basement steps

    Year-end statistics also included:

Admissions	1222	
Discharges	1225	
Deliveries	1203	
Abortions	57	(31 early; 19 intermediate; 7 late)
Undelivered	38	

    Calculate: Maternal death rate for the year.

2. Year-end discharge data for Cherub Hospital reveal:

Admissions	1353
Discharges (live):	
Delivered—live infant	1241
Delivered—aborted	63
Undelivered—antepartum	26
Undelivered—postpartum	19
Deaths (due to pregnancy)	2

    Calculate: Maternal death rate for the year.

3. Year-end obstetrical statistics include:

Admissions: 1582

Discharges:	*Live*	*Deaths*
Delivered of live infant	1495	3
Delivered of dead fetus	63	1
Undelivered—antepartum	14	0
Undelivered—postpartum	11	1

Calculate: Maternal death rate for the year, assuming all deaths were the result of conditions of pregnancy.

7. Fetal Death Rate (Stillborn Rate)

Although fetal deaths have already been mentioned, they have not been included in any of the computations carried out to this point. Remember that fetal deaths are *only* included in formulae specifically designated for them and that include the word *fetal* in them—fetal death rate, fetal autopsy rate. "Stillborn" and "aborted fetus" are terms commonly used to describe a fetal death. The criteria have already been mentioned as to what constitutes an early, intermediate, or late fetal death so they will not be reiterated here. Check for these designations earlier in this chapter. Remember that a fetus classified as a fetal death has not shown any signs of life upon entering the world (upon expulsion from the womb) and cannot be revived through any resuscitative means. Do not confuse newborn deaths with fetal deaths. If there is any sign of life at the time of birth, the birth is considered a live birth, even though death might occur shortly after delivery.

a. Included in Fetal Death Rates

Fetal death rates include only *intermediate* and *late* fetal deaths. This excludes fetuses of less than 20 weeks gestation or those weighing 500 grams or less. Early fetal deaths (500 grams or less in weight or less than 20 weeks gestation) are considered insufficiently developed to sustain life outside the womb.

b. Fetal Death Rate (Stillborn Rate)

Formula:

$$\frac{\text{Total number of intermediate and late fetal deaths for a period}}{\text{Total number of }births\text{ for the period}} \times 100$$

(including live births, and intermediate and late fetal deaths)

Note: This is another formula that does *not* use discharges in the denominator. The rationale for this is that every conceptus can be expelled (born) either dead or alive and the outcome is known at the moment of birth. By applying the "rate formula," and asking about the number of times something *could* happen, it becomes apparent that with each birth there is a chance the infant or fetus could be born with or without signs of life. Since only intermediate and late fetal deaths are included in a fetal death rate, they must also be included in the denominator (added to the live births) as well as in the numerator. If the term "births" is not specifically designated, keep in mind that "births" are also recorded as "newborn admissions."

Example: Newborn figures for April include a total of 505 live births. Live discharges included 515 newborns. Deaths included three newborn deaths, six early fetal deaths, four intermediate fetal deaths, and two late fetal deaths. To find the fetal death rate, add the number of intermediate and late fetal deaths (4 + 2 = 6) and divide by the number of live *births* plus the total intermediate and late fetal deaths (505 + 6 = 511), or 6 divided by 511, and then multiplied by 100, equals 1.17% [(6 ÷ 511) × 100].

SELF-TEST 26

Calculate the answers correctly to *two* decimal places.

1. A newborn unit recorded the following for May:

Admissions	238
Discharges (live)	235
Deaths (newborn)	1	(under 48 hours)
Fetal deaths	3	(1 early; 1 intermediate; 1 late)

    Calculate:

    a. Fetal death rate for May.

    b. Newborn death rate for May.

2. A newborn nursery's records for August reveal:

Bassinet count	18
Admissions	265
Discharges	260
Deaths	2
Fetal deaths	6

    (1 of 12-week gestation)
    (1 of 14-week gestation)
    (1 of 20-week gestation)
    (1 of 24-week gestation)
    (1 of 28-week gestation)
    (1 of 30-week gestation)

    Calculate:

    a. Fetal death rate for August.

    b. Newborn death rate for August.

3. October newborn data include:

Bassinet count	20
IP service days	565
Admissions	305
Discharges	311
Deaths	1
Fetal deaths	5

(1 weighed 465 gm)
(1 weighed 528 gm)
(1 weighed 936 gm)
(1 weighed 1001 gm)
(1 weighed 1055 gm)

Calculate:

a. Fetal death rate for October.

b. Newborn death rate for October.

C. SUMMARY

1. Inpatient deaths are those that occur during a patient's hospitalization as an inpatient, prior to discharge.
2. Outpatient deaths are those that occur
   a. in the emergency room before a person is admitted to the hospital.
   b. among outpatients who are series patients and come in routinely for treatment (chemotherapy, radiotherapy, rehabilitation, etc.) or for outpatient surgery.
   c. among home care patients or hospice patients seen routinely in their homes.
3. Deaths that are *not* included in routine death rates are
   a. outpatient deaths
   b. ER deaths
   c. DOAs
   d. fetal deaths
4. A&C deaths and NB deaths are combined and included together in the same death rate. They are not separated, as was done with census (admission) data.
5. A live birth is one that shows signs of life at the time of birth.
6. The term *fetal death* is preferred over the terms "stillborn," "abortion," or "aborted fetus."
7. The numerator in *all* death rates is the total number of deaths pertaining to that rate.
8. Helpful hints:
   a. Include only inpatient deaths—exclude OPs, DOAs, and fetal deaths.
   b. Death rates should be low.
   c. Death rates should be carried to two or three decimal places.
   d. The majority of death rates are computed by dividing the number of deaths by the number that were discharged.
   e. Net death rates exclude deaths that occur less than 48 hours after admission.

f.   Anesthesia death rates and maternal death rates should be extremely low and are generally figured only on a yearly basis.

g.   Fetal death rates include only intermediate and late fetal deaths.

9.   Gross Death Rate. Deaths divided by discharges.

10. Net Death Rate. (Total deaths minus those under 48 hours) divided by (total discharges minus deaths under 48 hours).

11. Newborn Death Rate. NB deaths divided by NB discharges.

12. Postoperative Death Rate. Postop deaths that occurred within ten days postop divided by the number of patients operated on.

13. Anesthesia Death Rate. Anesthesia deaths divided by the number of anesthetics administered.

14. Maternal Death Rate. Maternal (OB) deaths divided by OB discharges.

15. Fetal Death Rate. Intermediate and late fetal deaths divided by the total births (NB admissions) plus intermediate and late fetal deaths.

16. Maternal terms:

a.   Direct death—due to pregnancy.

b.   Indirect death—aggravated by pregnancy.

c.   Puerperium—a period of 42 days following delivery.

d.   Delivered—expelling contents of womb; may be single or multiple; may be live or dead.

e.   Undelivered—pregnancy-related admission, but the mother did not give birth during the admission.

f.   Synonymous terms: aborted; stillborn; fetal death.

g.   Partum—childbirth.

   1)   Antepartum—before childbirth.

   2)   Postpartum—after childbirth.

D. CHAPTER 5 TEST

Note: Compute all answers correctly to *two* decimal places.

1.   What is another name for stillborn?

2.   What is the gestational period for a/an

a.   early fetal death?

b.   intermediate fetal death?

c.   late fetal death?

3.   What is the gram weight for a/an

a.   early fetal death?

b.   intermediate fetal death?

c.   late fetal death?

4. Which IP deaths or those occurring during an inpatient hospitalization are *excluded* in each of the following death rates?
   a. Gross death rate

   b. Net death rate

   c. Fetal death rate

   d. Postop death rate

5. Which death rates *include* something other than discharges in the denominator? Indicate what is used in place of discharges.

6. Which death rate is also called an Institutional Death Rate?

7. Do most death rates separate NB from A&C?

8. Snowbird Hospital (May)—

		Deaths	
	Total	Under 48 hours	Over 48 hours
Deaths			
A&C	36	30	6
NB	5	1	4
Discharges (live)			
A&C	742		
NB	66		

   Calculate:
   a. Gross death rate.

   b. Net death rate.

9. Treetop Hospital—

Unit	Deaths	Discharges
Medical	25	310
Surgical	8	196
Pediatrics	2	38
OB	4	71
NB	1	80

   Calculate: Gross death rate.

10. During the month of July, the following surgical data was recorded:

Admissions	1015
Deaths	7 (less than 10 days postop = 2; more than 10 days postop = 5)
Discharges	997
Patients operated on	975
Surgical procedures	1018

    Calculate: Surgical postoperative death rate.

11. A maternal unit recorded the following data for August:

Maternal admissions	192
Discharges (live)	185
Deaths	1
Deliveries	181

    Calculate: Maternal death rate.

12. OB statistics for the year—

		OB Deaths
Admissions	2581	
Discharges:		
Delivered live newborn	2288	1
Delivered aborted (dead) fetus	239	1
Discharged undelivered	41	0

    Calculate: Maternal death rate.

13. Newborn statistics—

		< 48 hrs	*> 48 hrs*	*Early*	*Int.*	*Late*
NB births	235					
Discharges	228					
Deaths	4	3	1			
Fetal deaths	7			4	2	1

    Calculate: Newborn death rate.

14. Newborn statistics—

		< 48 hrs	> 48 hrs	Early	Int.	Late
NB births (live)	300					
Discharges	291					
Deaths	3	2	1			
Fetal deaths	26			18	5	3

Calculate:

a. Newborn death rate.

b. Fetal death rate.

15. Grant County Hospital (September)—

	Adm.	*Disch.*	*Deaths*	*< 48 hrs*	*> 48 hrs*
A&C	511	505	45	5	40
NB	83	80	1	0	1

Calculate:

a. Gross death rate.

b. Net death rate.

c. Newborn death rate.

16. Newborn statistics—

		Weeks Gestation
NB births (live)	86	
Discharges	75	
Deaths	2	
Fetal deaths	10	15, 18, 16, 28, 31, 25, 22, 14, 27, 20

Calculate:

a. Newborn death rate.

b. Fetal death rate.

17. General Surgery for June—

Admissions	354
Discharges	347
Patients operated on	334
Operations performed	372
Anesthesias administered	321
Deaths—Total	8
Postop	4 (3 less than 10 days postop)
Anesthesia	1

Calculate:

a. General surgery death rate.

b. Postop death rate for general surgery.

c. Anesthesia death rate for general surgery.

18. Woodland Hospital (July)—

	A&C	<48 hrs	>48 hrs	NB	<48 hrs	>48 hrs	E	I	L
Bed/bassinet count	225			20					
Admissions	1138			134					
Discharges (live)	1133			130					
Deaths	10	6	4	1	1	0			
IPSD	5722			503					
Fetal deaths							4	2	1

Calculate:

a. Gross death rate.

b. Net death rate.

c. NB death rate.

d. Fetal death rate.

19. Regional Hospital (March)—

Clinical Unit	Count Bed/Bass.		Adm.	IPSD	Live Disch.	Deaths	<48 hrs	>48 hrs	<10 hrs	>10 hrs
Medical	45		142	1280	135	8	5	3		
Surgical	20		81	518	72	5	2	3	4	1
Pediatric	8		66	188	58	1	0	1		
OB	18		118	495	114	1	0	1		
Neuropsych	10		44	261	38	2	1	1		
NB		15	110	466	105	2	1	1		
Totals	101	15	561	3208	522	19	9	10	4	1

Other Statistics:

						Deaths	<48 hrs	>48 hrs	<10 hrs	>10 hrs
Postop						4	2	2	3	1
Anesthesia						1				

Patients operated on	69
Anesthesias administered	77
Operations performed	99
Fetal deaths	9 (5 = early; 3 = intermediate; 1 = late)

Calculate:

a. Gross death rate.

b. Net death rate.

c. Newborn death rate.

d. Net medical service death rate.

e. Clinical service with the *lowest* gross death rate.

f. Clinical service with the *highest* gross death rate.

g. Postoperative death rate.

h. Anesthesia death rate.

i. Maternal death rate.

j. Fetal death rate.

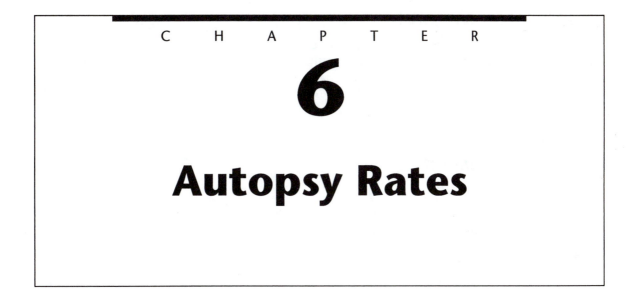

C H A P T E R

6

Autopsy Rates

CHAPTER OUTLINE

A. Terms/Information
1. Autopsy
2. Hospital Autopsy
3. Hospital Inpatient Autopsy
4. Coroner's/Medical Examiner's Cases
5. Who Performs an Autopsy
6. Hospital Autopsy

B. Autopsy Rates
1. Gross Autopsy Rate
2. Net Autopsy Rate
3. Hospital Autopsy Rate
4. Newborn Autopsy Rate
5. Fetal Autopsy Rate
C. Summary
D. Chapter 6 Test

LEARNING OBJECTIVES

After studying this chapter the learner should be able to:

1. Distinguish clearly between
   a. Autopsy vs. hospital autopsy vs. hospital inpatient autopsy.
   b. Net vs. gross autopsy.
2. Describe the types of deaths that most likely are "coroner's cases."
3. Describe when "coroner's cases" are included in hospital autopsies.

4. Distinguish which autopsies are included in hospital autopsies.
5. Compute the following autopsy rates:
   a. Gross
   b. Net
   c. Hospital
   d. Newborn
   e. Fetal

Autopsies are most commonly performed to determine the cause of death. Autopsies are also valuable learning tools for studying disease processes and to characterize the extent or type of changes wrought by disease and treatment. Hospital autopsies can improve clinical knowledge and can serve as a means of educating physicians.

An autopsy rate is a health care statistic that is often reported. It is the ratio of autopsies to deaths. Any patient who has expired is a candidate for an autopsy.

A. TERMS/INFORMATION

1. Autopsy

Inspection and partial dissection of a dead body to learn the cause of death, and the nature and extent of disease; a postmortem examination.

2. Hospital Autopsy

Postmortem examination performed by a hospital pathologist, or by a physician on the medical staff to whom the responsibility has been delegated, on the body of a person who has at some time been a hospital patient. The place where the examination is performed can vary.

3. Hospital Inpatient Autopsy

Postmortem examination performed in a hospital facility by a hospital pathologist, or by a physician on the medical staff to whom the responsibility has been delegated, on the body of a patient who died during inpatient hospitalization.

4. Coroner's/Medical Examiner's Cases

Specific kinds of deaths are reportable to the coroner's office. A coroner is an officer (often elected or appointed) who holds inquests regarding certain deaths, especially those considered violent, sudden, or unexplained.

Some jurisdictions employ a medical examiner, who is a physician officially authorized by a governmental unit (city or county) to ascertain causes of deaths, especially those not occurring under natural circumstances.

Throughout this book, the term *coroner's case* is used to designate cases handled by either the coroner or the medical examiner. Such cases meet the above criteria and are investigated by the coroner or medical examiner.

Hospitals encounter not only inpatient deaths but often outpatient deaths as well. Patients may be brought to the emergency room and expire there, or they may die during outpatient treatment (including surgery). Sometimes a hospital becomes involved with a home care patient who succumbs at home. An autopsy may be performed on these kinds of patients as well as those who are inpatients.

Coroner's cases require notification of the proper authorities (coroner or medical examiner). Cases of violence (such as murder, homicide, strangulation, suffocation, poisoning, gunshot wound) are coroner's cases, as are suicides, drownings, burns, etc. The investigation carried out by the coroner's office determines whether the death was accidental or the result of a crime.

Sudden deaths (in which the person was apparently in good health) or any other suspicious or unusual circumstances accompanying a death are also subject to investigation by the coroner. Also included are criminal or self-induced abortions or suspicious circumstances surrounding the birth of a stillborn infant. A patient who dies within 24 hours of admission to the hospital and who has not been under a physician's care for a disease, also becomes a coroner's case. Patients admitted to a hospital because of injuries that could have occurred because of violence or suicide and who die in the hospital become coroner's cases. Each state has laws governing which deaths are reportable to the coroner and must be investigated. Practitioners should familiarize themselves with these rules and regulations.

Unautopsied coroner's cases, as referred to in this text, are the bodies of deceased patients under the jurisdiction of the coroner that were not autopsied by the hospital pathologist or designated hospital physician.

5. *Who Performs an Autopsy*

In most hospitals, the pathologist performs an autopsy. If the death is a coroner's case and the coroner is not a medical examiner, the coroner contracts with a physician to perform this service. A physician (generally a pathologist) performs the autopsy, but the circumstances of the death are investigated by the coroner's office.

6. *Hospital Autopsy*

   a. *Who Performs*

   As stated in the definition, a hospital autopsy is performed by a member of the hospital's medical staff. The staff member is generally a pathologist, although another physician on the hospital's medical staff could be assigned to do the autopsy.

   b. *Where*

   Most hospitals have a morgue to which the dead bodies are taken at the time of death and it is here that most hospital autopsies are performed by the hospital pathologist. If onsite facilities are not provided, a designated place is generally specified for carrying out the autopsy.

   c. *Who Is Included*

   Any inpatient who expires could undergo an autopsy performed by the hospital pathologist. Since autopsies not only identify and establish the cause of death but also provide information that may be helpful in the future, it may also be advantageous to autopsy former patients who are not inpatients at the time of death. These could include ER deaths, outpatient deaths, home care deaths, or deaths of hospice patients. The term *hospital autopsy* can include outpatient as well as inpatient deaths. The formula for determining a hospital autopsy rate is the *only* formula in which outpatients are included with inpatient statistics.

   d. *Not Included*

   Fetal deaths are excluded from hospital autopsies. There is a special formula for computing a fetal autopsy rate. It has already been pointed out that fetal deaths and fetal autopsies are *never* included in any of the other statistical formulae.

   e. *Report Requirements*

   When an autopsy is performed by the hospital pathologist, an autopsy report must become a part of the patient's medical record. Tissue specimens from the patient must also be placed on file in the hospital.

f. **Legal Cases**

As previously mentioned, when some patients die they become coroner's cases and their bodies must be released to the proper authorities. If the autopsy is performed by the hospital pathologist, or by the physician delegated by the hospital to perform an autopsy, the case *is counted* as a hospital autopsy.

g. **Consent**

A physician obtains permission from the patient's next of kin to perform an autopsy. The autopsy is performed prior to the release of the body to the funeral home. Consent is not required for a coroner's case.

h. **Combine A&C/NB**

In autopsy rates—whether a hospital autopsy rate, gross autopsy rate, or net autopsy rate—the data on adults/children and newborns are combined, as is done when death rates are computed.

SELF-TEST 27

For each of the following examples, indicate whether the example is applicable to a *hospital autopsy* by answering yes or no.

1. Patient dies in the hospital. The body is autopsied by the hospital pathologist in the hospital morgue.   Yes   No

2. Patient dies in the hospital. The body is taken to the local morgue and the hospital pathologist performs the autopsy.   Yes   No

3. Patient dies in the hospital. The body is released to the medical examiner, who performs the autopsy.   Yes   No

4. Patient dies at home three weeks following inpatient discharge from the hospital. The body is brought to the hospital and the hospital pathologist performs an autopsy.   Yes   No

5. Three months after inpatient hospitalization, the patient is brought to the emergency room of the hospital, where he is pronounced DOA. The hospital pathologist performs an autopsy.   Yes   No

6. Patient is admitted to the hospital having received a stab wound to the abdomen. He expires during hospitalization and his body is released to the medical examiner, who performs the autopsy.   Yes   No

7. Patient is admitted to the hospital and dies four hours after admission. No sign of violence or suicide is present, but the patient had not been under a physician's care. The coroner removes the body and designates someone other than the hospital pathologist to perform the autopsy.   Yes   No

8. Patient is brought into the emergency room following a car accident and dies prior to inpatient admission. The coroner authorizes the hospital pathologist to perform the autopsy.   Yes   No

9. A cancer patient had been receiving cobalt therapy on an outpatient basis. Between scheduled outpatient visits, the patient died at home. The body was brought to the hospital, where the pathologist performed the autopsy.   Yes   No

10. The hospital pathologist is taking a two-week vacation and　　Yes　No
has a staff physician cover for him while he is gone. During
this time, a home care patient dies and the designated physician
does the autopsy.
11. A late fetal death is autopsied by the hospital pathologist.　　Yes　No

Note: Before starting to compute autopsy rates, consider carefully the data required. Since only those who have died will be autopsied, the denominator (those it *could* happen to) will be deaths, *not* discharges. The numerator will be the number of patients autopsied. Both numerator and denominator will generally be small numbers, but the percentage will be larger than death rates.

B. AUTOPSY RATES

1. Gross Autopsy Rate

Formula:

$$\frac{\text{Total autopsies performed on IP deaths for a period}}{\text{Total IP deaths}} \times 100$$

(Deaths include newborns as well as adults/children.)

Explanation: Remember that the term *gross* means *all*, with no subtractions or deletions of any cases.

Note: Only inpatients are included (not OPs). This rate indicates only the percentage of autopsies on IP deaths, irrespective of whether they were coroner's cases.

Example: During the first three months of the year, 18 inpatient deaths were recorded. Two of these were coroner's cases and fell under his jurisdiction. Of the remaining 16, an autopsy was performed on four patients. Four outpatient deaths were also reported and two of these were autopsied.

Since only inpatients are included in a *gross* autopsy rate, we can eliminate any reference to the outpatient data. Of the inpatients, four were autopsied and 18 inpatient deaths were recorded. Therefore, the gross autopsy rate is 4 divided by 18, then multiplied by 100, which yields a rate of 22.2% [(4 ÷ 18)] × 100). (*Note:* The two coroner's cases were included even though their bodies were not available for autopsy by the hospital pathologist.)

SELF TEST 28

Compute all rates correctly to *two* decimal places.

1. In November, one newborn death, eight adults/children deaths, and three intermediate/late fetal deaths were recorded. Three OP deaths were also recorded. A total of six autopsies were carried out by the hospital pathologist: one newborn, three adults/children, one late fetal death, one OP. Total discharges for the month were 331 adults/children and 67 newborns. Total admissions were 335 adults/children and 65 newborns.

   Calculate:

   a. Gross autopsy rate for November.

   b. * (R5) Gross death rate for November.

Note: For the remaining questions, the autopsies listed as coroner's cases are the unautopsied cases—the cases removed by the coroner for examination. The examination was not performed by the hospital pathologist or by a designated physician on the medical staff.

2. Pleasant Valley Hospital's first-quarter statistics included the following:

Inpatient:	A&C		NB	
Admissions	715		174	
Discharges	721		172	
Deaths (total)	16	(5 under 48 hrs)	2	(1 under 48 hrs)
Fetal deaths				
3 early				
2 intermediate				
1 late				
Autopsies	6		1	
Unautopsied (coroner)	2		1	

Calculate:

a. Gross autopsy rate.

b. * (R5) Gross death rate.

3. Silver City Hospital's last-quarter statistics contained the following information:

Inpatient:	A&C	NB
Admissions	1035	221
Discharges	1044	228
Deaths		
Under 48 hrs	11	2
Over 48 hrs	24	0
Autopsies (hospital)	18	1
Coroner's cases	5	1
Fetal deaths		

Fetal deaths		
Early	4	(no autopsies)
Intermediate	2	(1 autopsy)
Late	1	(coroner's case—not done by hospital pathologist)

Outpatient:		
Deaths	6	
Autopsies	5	(the death not included was a coroner's case)

Calculate:

a. Gross autopsy rate.

b. * (R5) Gross death rate.

c. * (R5) Fetal death rate.

2. Net Autopsy Rate

Formula:

$$\frac{\text{Total autopsies performed on IP deaths for a period}}{\text{Total IP deaths } \textit{minus} \text{ unautopsied cases released to legal authorities for the period}} \times 100$$

$$\frac{\text{Total IP autopsies for a given period}}{\text{Total IP deaths } \textit{minus} \text{ unautopsied coroners' cases}} \times 100$$

Explanation: Again, the use of the term *net* refers to the exclusion (subtraction) of certain patients. In this instance, they are the cases released to legal authorities (coroner/medical examiner), and thus are not available for hospital autopsy. Accordingly, they are subtracted from the total deaths. However, it must be noted that if the coroner authorizes the hospital pathologist to carry out the autopsy, it is included in the rate and is not subtracted. Subtract only those cases *unavailable* for autopsy by the hospital pathologist.

Note: No outpatients are included in a net autopsy rate; only inpatients are. Only the hospital autopsy rate includes available outpatients for computational purposes.

Example: Ten inpatient deaths are reported for March. Five of these deaths are autopsied by the hospital pathologist. Two are coroner's cases and the coroner requests that the hospital pathologist autopsy one of them.

A total of six deaths are autopsied by the hospital pathologist (one of which is a coroner's case that is included). The numerator contains these six cases. In the denominator, one case has to be subtracted from the total of ten deaths (since the coroner claimed one body, it was not available for autopsy), for a value of 9 (10 − 1). Dividing the numerator (6) by the denominator (9), and then multiplying by 100, gives a result of 66.7% [(6 ÷ 9) × 100].

Note: A net autopsy rate will be higher than a gross autopsy rate. The gross rate and the net rate have the same number in the numerator (6) but, by not subtracting the coroner's cases, there are 10 deaths rather than 9 in the denominator. With a lower number in the denominator the rate will be higher—in this case a net rate of 66.7% was found, in contrast to a gross rate of only 60%.

SELF-TEST 29

Rates are to be computed correctly to *two* decimal places.

1. Second-quarter statistics from General Hospital contained the following data:

Inpatients: Month	Deaths	Hospital Autopsy	Coroner's Cases
April	7	4	1
May	6	3	0
June	9	4	2

Outpatients: Month	Deaths	Hospital Autopsy	Coroner's Cases
April	3	2	1
May	4	2	1
June	5	2	2

Calculate:

a. Net autopsy rate for the period.

b. Gross autopsy rate for the period.

2. Happiness Hospital data for the period July through December was as follows:

Count: Bed count = 300   Bassinet count = 35

Inpatient:		A&C	NB
Admissions		1800	957
Discharges		1822	963
Deaths:			
Under 48 hrs		9	2
Over 48 hrs		23	2
Autopsies:		10	2
Coroner's cases		4	1

Fetal deaths:

Early	6	(none autopsied)
Intermediate	3	(2 autopsied; 1 taken by coroner)
Late	2	(1 autopsied; 1 taken by coroner)

Outpatient:

Deaths	8	
Autopsies	5	(two others were released to the coroner)

Calculate:

a. Net autopsy rate for the period.

b. * (R5) Net death rate for the period.

c. Gross autopsy rate for the period.

d. * (R5) Gross death rate for the period.

e. * (R5) Newborn death rate for the period.

f. * (R5) Fetal death rate for the period.

3. **Hospital Autopsy Rate (Adjusted)**

Formula:

$$\frac{\text{Number of } hospital \text{ autopsies for period}}{\text{Number of deaths of hospital patients whose bodies are available for hospital autopsy for that period}} \times 100$$

Note: In previous, formulae outpatients were *not* included along with inpatients. In calculating the hospital autopsy rate, OPs (outpatients) are included if their bodies were autopsied by the hospital pathologist or by a designated member of the medical staff.

Example: A hospital had 215 inpatient admissions in August and 205 discharges, of which 12 were deaths. Eight of these deaths were autopsied by the hospital pathologist. Two former patients died at home and were brought to the hospital and autopsied. To find the hospital autopsy rate, add all the hospital autopsies performed to determine the numerator (8 IP + 2 OP = 10 autopsies). The denominator contains all the inpatients who died (and could have been autopsied) during this same period (12) and the number of OP autopsied as well (2)—for a total of 14. The rate is determined by dividing 10 by 14, and then multiplying by 100, giving a hospital autopsy rate of 71.4% [(10 ÷ 14) × 100].

Example: In June, eight adults, one child, and one newborn died. A total of 240 admissions and 245 discharges were recorded in June. There were also two fetal deaths (one intermediate; one late). Autopsies were performed on four adults, the child, and the newborn, as well as the late fetal death. During June, one patient died in the ER and was autopsied, and two home care patients died and were taken to the hospital for autopsy.

To find the hospital autopsy rate, add the autopsies, except for the late fetal death [(4 + 1 + 1 = 6 IP) plus (1 + 2 = 3 OP), for a total of 6 + 3, which equals 9 autopsies]. Then add all the deaths on which autopsies could be performed [(8 + 1 + 1 = 10 IP) plus (1 + 2 = 3 OP), or 10 + 3 = 13]. Divide 9 by 13, and then multiply by 100. The result is a 69.2% hospital autopsy rate.

Note: Remember *never* include fetal death autopsies. Fetal deaths are only included in fetal rates—fetal death rates and fetal autopsy rates.

Computation Note: Autopsies listed as coroner's cases are the unautopsied cases—the cases removed by the coroner for examination. The examination was *not* performed by the hospital pathologist or by a designated physician on the medical staff, unless specifically indicated.

SELF-TEST 30

Compute all rates correctly to *two* decimal places.

1. A hospital with 250 beds recorded six deaths for the month of September. During this period there were 315 discharges of adults and children. The bassinet count was 18, and 95 newborns were discharged as well, with no newborn deaths recorded. The outpatient department recorded five outpatient deaths, two of which were reported from the emergency room. Autopsies were performed on three inpatients and three outpatients.

   Calculate:

   a. September hospital autopsy rate.

   b. Gross autopsy rate for September.

   c. * (R5) Gross death rate for September.

2. June statistics reveal the following:

	A&C	NB
IP admissions	475	75
IP discharges	472	72
IP deaths	9	1
IP autopsies	5	1
OP deaths	2	
OP autopsies	2	

Calculate:

a. June hospital autopsy rate.

b. Gross autopsy rate for June.

c. * (R5) Gross death rate for June.

3. May records indicate the following:

Inpatient Data

Admissions	A&C = 275	NB = 58
Discharges	A&C = 281	NB = 55

Deaths:

Adults	12	
Children	1	
Newborn	1	
Fetal	2	(both intermediate)

Autopsies:

Adults	6
Children	1
Newborn	1
Fetal	1

Outpatient Data

Deaths:

DOA	1	(which was autopsied)
ER	2	(one was autopsied and the other was taken by the coroner)
Home care	2	(one was autopsied)

Calculate:

a. Hospital autopsy rate for May.

b. Gross autopsy rate for May.

c. Net autopsy rate for May.

4. Out of a total of 441 discharges in June, seven were listed as deaths. Of these, three were autopsied by the hospital pathologist. Two were coroner's cases and, of these two, the coroner requested that the hospital pathologist perform one of the autopsies, which he did. Three outpatients also died, but only two were autopsied by the pathologist. The third was removed from the hospital by the coroner.

Calculate:

a. June hospital autopsy rate.

b. Gross autopsy rate for June.

c. Net autopsy rate for June.

4. *Newborn Autopsy Rate*

Formula:

$$\frac{\text{Autopsies performed on NB deaths for a period}}{\text{Total NB deaths for the period}} \times 100$$

Example: Seventy-four births occurred during the month of July, and a total of 72 newborns were discharged. One newborn expired shortly after birth. Five fetal deaths were also reported during July—three were intermediate fetal deaths and two were late fetal deaths. An autopsy was performed on the NB death and three of the fetal deaths (one intermediate and two late).

Applying the formula, and excluding any reference to the fetal deaths or autopsies, leaves only one newborn autopsied (only one newborn died). This results in a 100% newborn autopsy rate for July (1 divided by 1, and then multiplied by 100, equals 100%).

SELF-TEST 31

Compute all rates correctly to *two* decimal places.

1. Newborn figures for October:

Admissions	223	
Discharges	225	
Deaths	2	
Autopsies	1	
Fetal deaths	5	(2 early; 2 intermediate; 1 late)
Fetal autopsies	1	(done only on the late death)

    Calculate:

    a. Newborn autopsy rate for October.

    b. * (R5) Newborn death rate for October.

2. A neonatal unit records two newborn deaths and two term infants who were stillborn. An autopsy is performed on the two newborns and one of the stillborns. A total of 315 newborns were born, and 312 were discharged during the same month.

   Calculate: Newborn autopsy rate for the month.

3. Out of 211 discharges, a neonatal unit had one death, which was autopsied by the hospital pathologist. A mother delivered in a taxicab on the way to the hospital, and she and the infant were admitted upon arrival at the hospital, but the baby died shortly after admission. An autopsy was performed on this infant as well.

   Calculate: Newborn autopsy rate for the period.

5. Fetal Autopsy Rate

Formula:

$$\frac{\text{Autopsies performed on intermediate and late fetal deaths for a period}}{\text{Total intermediate and late fetal deaths for period}} \times 100$$

Example: Ten fetal deaths were logged by the obstetric unit, of which four were early fetal deaths, four were intermediate fetal deaths, and two were late fetal deaths. Of these, the two late fetal deaths were autopsied.

Since only intermediate and late fetal deaths are included in the fetal autopsy rate and both autopsies were performed on late fetal deaths, the number 2 is placed in the numerator and the number 6 in the denominator (4 intermediate + 2 late fetal deaths). Dividing 2 by 6, and then multiplying by 100, gives a fetal autopsy rate of 33.3% [(2 ÷ 6) × 100].

SELF-TEST 32

Compute all rates correctly to *two* decimal places.

1. Five fetal deaths were recorded in January. Also recorded were 233 live births and 240 live newborn discharges. One newborn death was also recorded. Three fetal deaths were early deaths and two were intermediate fetal deaths, one of which was autopsied, as was the newborn death.

   Calculate:

   a. Fetal autopsy rate for January.

   b. Newborn autopsy rate for January.

   c. * (R5) Fetal death rate for January.

   d. * (R5) Newborn death rate for January.

2. In December, ten fetal deaths were reported. One of these was a stillborn term infant. Of the remaining, one was a late fetal death and two were intermediate fetal deaths; the others were early fetal deaths. One intermediate fetal death was of a suspicious nature and was removed by the coroner. Of the remaining fetal deaths, an autopsy was performed on the stillborn and late fetal death by the hospital pathologist. A total of 351 live births, 348 live newborn dis-

charges, and one newborn death (which was not autopsied) were recorded in December.

Calculate:

a. Fetal autopsy rate for December.

b. * (R5) Fetal death rate for December.

c. Newborn autopsy rate for December.

d. * (R5) Newborn death rate for December.

C. SUMMARY

1. A hospital autopsy is performed by a physician who is designated by the hospital, most commonly the hospital pathologist.
2. Patients *included* are hospital inpatients autopsied by a designated medical staff physician. Hospital outpatients also are included, but only in the rate referred to as "hospital autopsy rate," as long as the outpatients were autopsied by the designated physician.
3. *Excluded* are fetal death autopsies. These are used only in a fetal autopsy rate.
4. Outpatient autopsies are included only in a hospital autopsy rate.
5. A&C and NB are combined and included together in most autopsy rates.
6. Coroner's cases (medical examiner's cases) include those bodies that need to be investigated further to rule out foul play. They include the cases that fall under his/her jurisdiction—most commonly they involve violence or deaths that are suspicious in nature. Cases may include drownings, poisonings, or burns, as well as abortions.
7. If the case is a coroner's case and the autopsy is performed by the hospital pathologist, it is included as a hospital autopsy.
8. The numerator in all autopsy rates is the total number of autopsies performed that are related to the specific autopsy rate.
9. The denominator in autopsy rates is always comprised of deaths, although some deaths may be excluded in certain rates.
10. In general, autopsy rates are computed by dividing the number of autopsies by the number of deaths.
11. Hospital Autopsy Rate: IP and OP autopsies divided by deaths of hospital patients whose bodies are available for hospital autopsy.
12. Newborn Autopsy Rate: NB autopsies divided by NB deaths.
13. Fetal Autopsy Rate: Intermediate and late fetal autopsies divided by the intermediate and late fetal deaths.
14. Gross Autopsy Rate: IP autopsies divided by IP deaths.
15. Net Autopsy Rate: IP autopsies divided by IP deaths minus the unautopsied coroner's cases.

D. CHAPTER 6 TEST

1. Which autopsy rate may include outpatients as well as inpatients?

2. Who is authorized to perform a hospital autopsy?

3. What types of death fall under the jurisdiction of the coroner?

4. Which deaths, even though autopsied, are *excluded* in hospital autopsy rates?

5. Do autopsy rates combine A&C and NB autopsies or are they maintained separately?

6. Is a body that has been autopsied by the medical examiner included in a hospital autopsy rate if the medical examiner is not on the hospital medical staff?

7. What is excluded in a net autopsy rate that is included in a gross autopsy rate?

Note: All computations should be correct to *two* decimal places.

8. Snowmass Hospital (June)

		Autopsies		
	Deaths	**Yes (HP)***	**No**	**Coroner**
Inpatient	39	5	32	2
Outpatient	2	2		

Calculate:

a. Gross autopsy rate.

b. Net autopsy rate.

c. Hospital autopsy rate.

9. Gossamer Hospital (February)

A&C	**NB**	
Beds/bassinets	250	30
Admissions	1210	205
Discharges	1210	200
Deaths 14	2	
Autopsies:		
Yes (HP)	5	1
No 7	0	
Coroner	2	1
IPSD 6252	701	

*HP=Hospital Pathologist

Calculate:

    a. NB autopsy rate.

    b. A&C autopsy rate.

    c. Gross autopsy rate.

    d. Net autopsy rate.

    e. * (R4) Percentage of bed occupancy for A&C.

    f. * (R4) Percentage of bassinet occupancy for NB.

10. Crestline Hospital (May)

IP:	A&C	NB	Fetal Deaths		
			Early	Int.	Late
Admissions	850	175			
Discharges	839	168			
Deaths	13	1	5	2	1
Autopsies					
Yes (HP)	5	1	0	1	1
No	7	0	4	1	0
Coroner	1	0	1	0	0

OP:	Deaths	Autopsies		
		Yes (HP)	No	Coroner
DOA	6	2	2	2
ER	2	1	0	1
HC	2	1	1	0

Calculate:

a. Gross autopsy rate.

b. Net autopsy rate.

c. Hospital autopsy rate.

d. Fetal autopsy rate.

e. Newborn autopsy rate.

11. Riverside Hospital

| | Admissions | | Discharges | | Deaths | | Autopsies | | | | | |
| | | | | | | | A&C | | | NB | | |
	A&C	NB	A&C	NB	A&C	NB	Yes	No	Cor.	Yes	No	Cor.
Jan.	801	165	797	162	11	3	3	7	1	1	2	0
Feb.	788	151	775	146	9	1	2	6	1	1	0	0
Mar.	818	161	801	157	15	2	4	9	2	1	0	1

Calculate:

a. Gross autopsy rate for the entire period.

b. Net autopsy rate for the entire period.

c. Newborn autopsy rate for the entire period.

d. January gross autopsy rate.

e. February net autopsy rate.

f. March newborn autopsy rate.

12. Valley View Hospital (August)

| | | | | Autopsies | | |
Patient Care Units	Adm.	Disch.	Deaths	Yes (HP)	No	Coroner
Medical	467	461	27	8	18	1
Surgical	102	98	5	2	2	1
Pediatrics	70	65	1	1	0	0
OB	332	330	1	1	0	0
GYN	65	62	0	0	0	0
Orthopedics	63	65	1	0	1	0
Neurology	26	27	3	2	0	1
NB	277	275	1	0	1	0
Totals	1402	1383	39	14	22	3

Calculate:

a. Newborn autopsy rate.

b. Gross autopsy rate.

c. Net autopsy rate.

d. Net medical unit autopsy rate.

e. Gross surgical unit autopsy rate.

7

Length of Stay/ Discharge Days

CHAPTER OUTLINE

A. Terms
1. Length of Stay (LOS)
2. Total Length of Stay
3. Discharge Days (DD)
4. Average Length of Stay
B. Calculating Length of Stay
1. General
2. A&D Same Day
3. Admitted One Day and Discharged the Next

4. Longer Stays
C. Total Length of Stay
1. Importance of Discharge Days
2. Totaling
D. Average Length of Stay
1. Adults and Children (A&C)
2. Newborn (NB)
E. Day on Leave of Absence
F. Summary
G. Chapter 7 Test

LEARNING OBJECTIVES

After studying this chapter the learner should be able to:

1. Define "length of stay."
2. Define "discharge days."
3. Identify the days counted and excluded in LOS determinations.
4. Describe when discharge days are acquired.
5. Describe when a "leave of absence" day is acquired.

6. Identify the formulae in which a leave of absence day is counted and when it is excluded.
7. Compute the following for A&C and NB:
   a. Individual lengths of stay.
   b. Total lengths of stay for a designated period.
   c. Average length of stay.

In the chapter on census, reference was made to inpatient service days, which are based on admission data—(data that pertains to all patients who receive service in a hospital on a specific day). In this chapter, computation will be based on discharge data, and the term *discharge day(s)* is used to distinguish these days from those based on admission data. Service days accumulate on a daily basis and a total is derived each day. Discharge days are compiled at the time of discharge and are not recorded until the patient is discharged from the hospital. As long as a patient is hospitalized, there will be *no* discharge days for that patient, because discharge days are compiled only *after* the patient is discharged from the hospital.

At the time of discharge (or death), a "length of stay" (LOS) is determined for each patient. This represents the number of days the patient was hospitalized and received service in the hospital. Synonymous terms include (inpatient) "days of stay," "duration of hospitalization," or "discharge days."

A. TERMS

1. Length of Stay (LOS) (For One Inpatient):

The number of calendar days from admission to discharge.

2. Total Length of Stay (For All Inpatients):

The sum of the days of stay of any group of inpatients discharged during a specified period of time.

3. Discharge Days (DD):

Same as Length of Stay or Total Length of Stay (see above).

4. Average Length of Stay:

The average length of hospitalization of a group of inpatients discharged during the period under consideration.

B. CALCULATING LENGTH OF STAY

Certain rules apply, including the following:

1. General

Each day counts as a discharge day *except* the day of discharge. In general, the patient's day of admission is counted as one day, as are all intervening days between admission and discharge, but *not* the day of discharge.

Example: A patient is admitted on June 3 and discharged on June 10. The patient has a length of stay of seven days, counting June 3, 4, 5, 6, 7, 8, 9 but *not* June 10. Notice that the length of stay can be determined by subtracting the date of admission from the date of discharge when the patient has been admitted and discharged during the same month (subtract 3 from 10 to obtain a length of stay of 7 days).

Example: The length of stay of a patient admitted one month and discharged the following month is computed in a similar fashion. If a patient is admitted on May 28 and discharged on June 4, the May figure is subtracted from the number of days in May (31) and added to the number of days the patient was hospitalized in June (4), resulting in a length of stay of 7 days ($31 - 28 = 3 + 4 = 7$). Keep in mind, however, the rule of not counting the day of discharge. The days that are counted are May 28, 29,

30, 31, June 1, 2, 3—for a total of 7 days. The final figure arrived at is identical when you use either method of computation, but it is important to remember the rule regarding which days are actually counted.

2. A&D Same Day

Any patient admitted and discharged on the same day accumulates a length of stay of *one* day. No patient admitted to the hospital ever has 0 (zero) days or negative days credited as a length of stay. Therefore, the patient is credited with a one-day length of stay even if the patient was admitted at 6:00 A.M. and discharged (or perhaps transferred to another hospital) at 8:00 A.M..

Example: A patient admitted at 10:00 A.M. on April 2 and discharged at 6:00 P.M. on April 2 acquires a length of stay of one day.

3. Admitted One Day and Discharged the Next

A patient who is admitted one day and discharged the following day also is credited with a length of stay of *one* day.

Example: A patient admitted at 9:00 P.M. on March 5 and discharged the following day at 2:00 P.M. has a length of stay of one day.

4. Longer Stays

For longer stays, the general rule of counting the day of admission and all subsequent days *except* the day of discharge applies.

Examples:

a. Same Month: A patient is admitted on December 1 and discharged December 13. The length of stay for that admission is 12 days. Officially, the days counted are December 1, 2, 3, 4, 5, 6, 7, 8, 9, 10, 11, 12, but not December 13, and the total is 12 days. Unofficially, subtract 1 from 13, which also gives a total of 12 days.

b. Adjacent Months: A patient admitted on February 28 and discharged on March 2 has a total length of stay of two days. (Count February 28 and March 1, but not March 2). Unofficially, 28 − 28 = 0 + 2 = 2. It is important to be accurate and to double-check the totals.

Another Example: A patient is admitted on March 30 and discharged on May 5. In this instance, one must add the days in April (30) to the March and May figures. The total includes two days in March (30, 31) plus the 30 days in April plus four days in May (1, 2, 3, 4), for a total of 36 days. Alternatively, subtract 30 from 31 (1), add in the 30 days in April, and then add five days in May, which gives the same total as before— 36 days.

c. Adjacent Years: A patient is admitted on December 28, 1988 and discharged on January 4, 1989. The total length of stay is 7 days (December 28, 29, 30, 31 plus January 1, 2, 3).

Another Example: In long-term care facilities patients may be residents for longer than a year. A patient admitted on November 11, 1987 and discharged (or who expired) on January 10, 1989 has a length of stay of 426 days. For November 1987 the total is 20 days; add the December total of 31 days; add to that the total days in 1988, 366 days (a leap year); add the January 1989 total of 9 days; and the result is a total of 426 days (20 + 31 + 366 + 9 = 426).

SELF-TEST 33

Compute the length of stay for the following patients. (In questions 1 through 6, assume that the dates are in the same year and that it is a non-leap year.)

1. Admitted 5-25   Discharged 5-25   _____
2. Admitted 5-15   Discharged 5-16   _____
3. Admitted 5-11   Discharged 5-25   _____
4. Admitted 5-27   Discharged 6-3   _____
5. Admitted 5-31   Discharged 6-2   _____
6. Admitted 5-29   Discharged 7-5   _____
7. Admitted 12-26-88   Discharged 1-10-89   _____
8. Admitted 12-22-88   Discharged 3-7-89   _____
9. Admitted 11-19-87   Discharged 3-17-88   _____
10. Admitted 10-31-87   Discharged 4-5-89   _____

C. TOTAL LENGTH OF STAY

The total length of stay for all patients during a specified period is commonly referred to as *discharge days*. In computing census data, the total is stated in terms of service days, but here the total length of stay is most commonly referred to as discharge days. Remember that no discharge days are compiled until the patient is discharged, so a patient who has been hospitalized for six months and is still an inpatient has *no* discharge days, even though the patient has received six months of service. Service days are credited daily, discharge days only upon discharge. A patient who is hospitalized for more than a year will have all the discharge days credited on the day of discharge (for instance, 702 days if the patient is hospitalized from 2-3-87 until 1-5-89). Therefore, it should be noted that service days and discharge days—even though often similar in number—are *not* interchangeable.

1. Importance of Discharge Days

Discharge days are important in analyzing and comparing patient subgroups in terms of diseases, treatment, age, and so on. For instance, if a patient is admitted to the hospital for an uncomplicated appendectomy and the length of stay computes to 14 days, there is reason to check further because most appendectomy patients are discharged in under five days. In addition, it may be that only the patients of certain doctors have longer than normal lengths of stay for their diagnoses and the medical staff may choose to take this under advisement. Discharge days are used to compute the average length of stay and this, in turn, may serve as the basis for comparing various subgroups.

2. Totaling

Various totals may be requested.

Example: Five patients are discharged on July 4. The individual lengths of stay are 10 days, 5 days, 3 days, 8 days, and 2 days. The total discharge days for patients discharged on July 4 is 28 days.

Example: The following patients were discharged on March 1:

Name	Age	Clinical Service	Length of Stay
Adams, A.	50	Medical	12 days
Baker, B.	23	Surgical	5 days
Carter, C.	8	Medical	22 days
Davis, D.	22	Obstetrical	3 days
Eaton, E.	8	Pediatrics	3 days
Fisher, F.	35	Surgical	7 days
Grant, G.	80	Medical	27 days
Hanson, H.	73	Medical	9 days
Irwin, I.	13	Pediatrics	4 days
Jones, J.	59	Medical	8 days

The total length of stay (discharge days) for all patients on March 1 is 100.

If the requirement is to total the length of stay for each clinical service, the results would be:

Medical	78 days	5 patients (12 + 22 + 27 + 9 + 8)
Surgical	12 days	2 patients (5 + 7)
Obstetrics	3 days	1 patient (3)
Pediatrics	7 days	2 patients (3 + 4)

If the requirement is to find the length of stay based on the ages of patients by decade, the results would be:

0 through 9	3 days	1 patient (3)
10 through 19	4 days	1 patient (4)
20 through 29	8 days	2 patients (5 + 3)
30 through 39	7 days	1 patient (7)
40 through 49	—	0
50 through 59	20 days	2 patients (12 + 8)
60 through 69	22 days	1 patient
70 through 79	9 days	1 patient
80 through 89	27 days	1 patient (27)
90 through 99	—	0

D. AVERAGE LENGTH OF STAY

Since totals alone do not give us much information that is useful, the most common use of discharge days is in determining the average length of stay. An average is usually much more easily interpreted, both for statistical purposes and for comparisons. The average length of stay is used to give a representation of the average duration of hospitalization of a group.

1. Adults and Children (A&C)

When calculating the average length of stay, the adults and children average is computed separately from that of newborns. The formulas are identical in their computation method, but each of the two groups is calculated separately. When a question asks for average length of stay, it is assumed that the average for A&C is to be determined and not the combination of adults and children and newborns.

Formula:

$$\frac{\text{Total length of stay (discharge days)}}{\text{Total discharges}}$$

(*Note:* Include length of stays for deceased patients but exclude NBs from this formula.)

Example: If a hospital had a total of 700 discharges during the month of March, with a total of 3500 discharge days (DD), the numbers alone are not very significant. However, by stating that the average length of stay of inpatients during March was five days, we have a much more significant statistic. This is determined by placing the discharge days (3500) in the numerator and dividing by the total number of patients discharged (700), resulting in an average length of stay of five days (3500 divided by 700 = 5 days).

Example: The discharges for the first quarter of the year for obstetrical patients totaled 275. The total discharge days, for the same quarter, of OB patients was 825. To compute the average length of stay of OB patients during the first quarter of the year, divide 825 by 275, which results in an average length of stay of 3 days.

Note: Newborns are again *excluded* in general length of stay computations, as they were in determining bed occupancy. Newborns generally are hospitalized the same length of time as their mothers (who are OB patients). Compared to other types of illnesses and disorders, this is most commonly a short stay. By including both mothers and babies in the determination of average length of stay for all patients, the average becomes distorted, resulting in a shorter length of stay and not representative of all lengths of stay. OB patients are included in the adults and children (A&C) length of stay, but newborns (NB) are excluded and kept separate. The formula for determination of newborn average length of stay is stated in the next section of this chapter. The newborn average length of stay is determined in the same manner as that of adults and children average length of stay.

SELF-TEST 34

1. Data for January:

	A&C	NB
Bed/bassinet count	50	5
Admissions	140	35
Discharges	143	36
IP service days	1203	138
Discharge days	1001	108

Determine:

a. Average length of stay for adults and children (A&C) in January.

b. Average length of stay for newborns in January.

c. Average length of stay for the all inpatients (A&C plus NB) in January.

2. November Data:

	A&C	*NB*
Bed/bassinet count	100	8
Admissions	345	89
Discharges	338	102
IP service days	2765	215
Discharge days	2724	225

Determine:

a. Average length of stay (A&C) for November.

b. Average length of stay for newborns in November.

3. The following patients are discharged on June 10:

	Admitted	*Discharged*	*Service*
Abbott, A.	5-16	6-10	Medical
Black, B.	5-31	6-10	Surgical
Canfield, C.	6-06	6-10	Medical
Draper, D.	6-10	6-10	Medical
Eckhart, E.	6-02	6-10	Surgical
Franke, F.	6-08	6-10	Obstetrics
Graber, G.	6-09	6-10	Medical
Huber, H.	5-30	6-10	Surgical
Ibsen, I.	4-30	6-10	Medical
James, J.	6-07	6-10	Obstetrics

Determine:

a. Average length of stay for June 10.

b. Average length of stay for medical patients on June 10.

c. Average length of stay for surgical patients on June 10.

d. Average length of stay for obstetrical patients on June 10.

4. February statistics:
   Bed count: 125
   Bassinet count: 12

Service	Adm.	Dis. (Live)	Deaths	IPSD	DD
Medical	300	303	6	1500	1516
Surgical	120	124	3	960	972
Obstetrics	72	68	1	195	202
Pediatrics	63	65	1	188	194
Newborn	62	65	1	153	165

Determine:

a. Average length of stay (A&C).

b. Average length of stay of medical patients in February.

c. Average length of stay of surgical patients in February.

d. Average length of stay of obstetrical patients in February.

e. Average length of stay of pediatric patients in February.

f. Average length of stay of newborns in February.

g. * (R4) IP bed occupancy percentage for February.

h. * (R4) Bassinet occupancy percentage for February.

5. Quarterly statistics:

	Jan.–Mar.	Apr.–June	July–Sept.	Oct.–Dec.
Admissions	1800	1715	1913	1888
Discharges	1785	1717	1902	1885
IP service days	9013	8621	9589	9461
Discharge days	8955	8581	9502	9470

Determine:

a. Average length of stay for the year.

b. Quarter with the lowest average length of stay.

c. Quarter with the highest average length of stay.

6. A 40-bed surgical unit records the following data for the year:

Type of Surgery	Adm.	Dis. (Live)	Deaths	IPSD	DD
EENT	228	225	1	483	490
Neurosurgery	112	115	7	1123	1133
Thoracic	202	205	3	1676	1682
Abdominal	1010	1006	12	8012	7095
GU	276	275	2	1659	1654
Other	128	126	1	557	537

Determine:

a. Average length of stay for patients on the surgical unit for the year.

b. Surgical unit that had the highest average length of stay for the year.

c. Surgical unit with the lowest average length of stay for the year.

d. Average length of stay for patients on each surgical unit.

2. Newborn (NB)

Formula:

$$\frac{\text{Total newborn length of stay (discharge days)}}{\text{Total newborn discharges}}$$

(Remember that newborns who expired after birth are included in this formula.)

Example: A newborn unit recorded the following data during February: 135 births, 140 discharges, 510 newborn service days, and 560 newborn discharge days. To compute the average newborn length of stay, divide 560 (DD) by 140 (total newborn discharges), which results in an average NB length of stay of 4 days.

SELF-TEST 35

1. A newborn nursery records the following statistics for July:

Bassinet count	15
Admissions	204
NB service days	408
Discharges	201
NB discharge days	420

Determine:

a. Average length of stay for newborns in July.

b. * (R4) Percentage of occupancy for the NB nursery in July.

2. A 10-bed NB nursery reports the following for October 1 through October 10:

	10-1	10-2	10-3	10-4	10-5	10-6	10-7	10-8	10-9	10-10
Births	3	2	4	1	1	2	3	3	1	2
Discharges	2	3	5	2	1	1	2	3	2	0
IPSD	8	6	6	5	6	7	5	4	6	5
Discharge days	7	8	10	6	4	5	4	5	6	0

Determine:

a. Average newborn length of stay for October 1 through October 10.

b. Average newborn length of stay for October 1 through October 5.

c. Average newborn length of stay for October 6 through October 10.

d. * (R4) Average newborn occupancy percentage for the entire period (October 1 through October 10).

e. * (R4) Average NB occupancy percentage for October 1 through October 5.

f. * (R4) Average NB occupancy percentage for October 6 through October 10.

3. A newborn nursery records the following data for January 15:

	NB	Birthweight		Mother
Admissions:	girl	7 lb	6 oz	Arends, A.
	girl	6 lb	10 oz	Brady, B.
	boy	9 lb	1 oz	Clark, C.
	boy	8 lb	3 oz	Doran, D.
	girl	5 lb	11 oz	Eaton, E.
	girl	8 lb	1 oz	Flack, F.

	NB	Born	Discharged	Mother
Discharges:	girl	1-13	1-15	Good, G.
	boy	1-12	1-15	Hart, H.
	girl	1-14	1-15	Ivey, I.
	girl	1-10	1-15	Juhl, J.
	boy	1-13	1-15	King, K.

Determine:

a. Average length of stay for newborns discharged on January 15.

b. Average length of stay for boys discharged on January 15.

c. Average length of stay for girls discharged on January 15.

d. Average birth weight of newborns born on January 15.

    e.   Average birth weight of newborn boys born on January 15.

    f.   Average birth weight of newborn girls born on January 15.

E. DAY ON LEAVE OF ABSENCE

A day occurring after the admission and prior to the discharge of a hospital inpatient, when the patient is *not* present at the census-taking hour because he or she is on leave of absence from the hospital.

    A leave of absence is an absence authorized by the patient's physician. Some patients are given passes to leave the hospital, generally for a home visit (often to see how well they can manage at home prior to discharge) or to take care of important business. A leave of absence generally involves an overnight pass, and therefore the patient would not be on the clinical unit at the CTT (census-taking time). Weekend passes may also be granted, often with the patient allowed to leave on Friday evening and return to the hospital on Sunday evening. These absences will exclude the patient from the inpatient census data. Only leaves that involve at least 24 hours of absence are considered in compiling statistical data.

    Leave of absence days differ from a discharge and readmission. A leave of absence is a segment of an uninterrupted hospitalization, whereas in the latter instance the patient may be discharged one day and readmitted for the same or a different diagnosis the next day. This latter scenario is not considered a leave of absence day.

    There is no uniform policy among hospitals regarding the use of leave of absence days and the final decision is up to the patient's attending physician. Facilities that admit patients for longer stays, such as rehabilitation facilities, mental hospitals, nursing homes, and long-term drug treatment centers, are most apt to grant a leave of absence. Patients in such facilities may need gradual reorientation to total self-care and their length of time away from the facility may begin with a leave of absence of a day or weekend and then gradually increase prior to final discharge.

    The use of leave of absence days affects the compilation of statistical data. The formulae in which the leave of absence day is *included* for statistical purposes is as follows:

1. *Discharge Days*—A patient accumulates a discharge day during the time the patient is on a leave of absence (one discharge day for each day on leave of absence).
2. *Average Length of Stay*—Since this is based on the discharge days, the leave of absence day is also included in compiling the average length of stay.

Leave of absence days are *excluded* in determining or computing the following statistics:

1. *Inpatient Service Days*—No service is being rendered the patient during the patient's absence from the hospital.
2. *Inpatient Census*—The patient is not included in the census at the census-taking hour.
3. *Bed Occupancy Percentage*—Since IPSD are used to determine the percentage of bed occupancy, the patient is not included as a patient who is occupying a bed while he or she is on leave of absence.

F. SUMMARY

1. Length of stay (LOS) or discharge days (DD) refer to the number of days the patient was hospitalized (from admission to discharge).

2. LOS or DD accumulate only upon discharge from the hospital.
3. All days are counted in determining LOS, except the day of discharge, unless the patient was admitted and discharged on the same day, in which case a LOS of one day is recorded.
4. To calculate the LOS, subtract the date of admission from the date of discharge.
5. Total daily discharge days are the sum of all LOS of patients discharged on a specific date.
6. Average LOS is the total length of stays of all patients discharged during a specified period of time divided by the total number of discharges during that specified period.
7. A&C and NB data should be kept separate. Generally the two are *not* combined, especially when calculating the average length of stay.
8. A leave of absence day is granted prior to discharge, and the day is *included* (counted) in computing
   a. discharge days
   b. average length of stay
   However, it is *excluded* in computing
   a. IPSD
   b. IP census
   c. bed occupancy percentage

G. CHAPTER 7 TEST

Note: Answers should be correct to *two* decimal places.

1. When does a patient acquire discharge days?

2. Is it possible to have over 365 discharge days? If so, when?

3. What numbers are totaled to determine discharge days?

4. In figuring the length of stay for a patient who is hospitalized for more than one day—
   a. Is the day of admission counted as a discharge day? Yes   No
   b. Is the day of discharge counted as a discharge day? Yes   No

5. How does a patient acquire a leave of absence day?

6. a. In which formulae is a leave of absence day included in the computation?

   b. In which formulae is a leave of absence day excluded?

7. Under what circumstances would a patient not have any discharge days at the end of the year?

8. Determine the lengths of stay for each of the following, assuming the dates occur in a non-leap year:
   a. Admitted 8-03   Discharged 8-04   _____
   b. Admitted 8-15   Discharged 8-15   _____
   c. Admitted 12-01   Discharged 2-08   _____
   d. Admitted 8-02   Discharged 8-20   _____

e.   Admitted 3-24   Discharged 4-04   _____

f.   Admitted 5-12   Discharged 11-30   _____

g.   Admitted 2-28   Discharged 3-07   _____

h.   Admitted 3-29   Discharged 4-01   _____

i.   Admitted 6-02-89   Discharged 7-04-90   _____

9. Healthful Hospital (April)

	A&C	*NB*
Bed/Bassinet count	180	15
Admissions	905	88
Discharges	895	86
Deaths	7	1
Autopsies:		
Yes (HP)	3	1
No	3	0
Coroner's case	1	0
IPSD	4820	339
Discharge days	4785	330

Calculate:

a.   Average length of stay for A&C.

b.   Average length of stay for NB.

c.   * (R5) Gross death rate.

d.   * (R6) Gross autopsy rate.

e.   * (R4) Percentage of occupancy for A&C.

f.   * (R4) Percentage of occupancy for NB.

10. Hopeful Hospital—Discharge List for June 3.

Live Discharges	*Service*	*Date of Admission*	*Date of Discharge*	*LOS*
A. Adams	Surgical	5-31	6-3	
B. Brown	Medical	5-19	6-3	
C. Clark	Surgical	5-23	6-3	
D. Davis	Psychiatric	5-03	6-3	
E. Edgar	OB	5-31	6-3	
G. Edgar	NB	5-31	6-3	
H. Horn	OB	5-28	6-3	
J. Jones	Orthopedic	5-24	6-3	
K. King	Urology	5-28	6-3	

Live Discharges	Service	Date of Admission	Date of Discharge	LOS
L. Long	ENT	6-02	6-3	
M. Mason	Gynecology	6-03	6-3	
N. Norris	Medical	5-29	6-3	
O. Olson	Urology	5-30	6-3	
P. Parks	Gynecology	5-27	6-3	

Deaths

R. Rill	Medical	5-29	6-3	

Calculate:

    a.   Length of stay for each of the above discharges.

    b.   Average length of stay for A&C.

    c.   Average length of stay for NB.

    d.   Average LOS for medical patients.

    e.   Average LOS for surgical patients.

    f.   Average LOS for urological patients.

11. Hillside Medical Center (October)
    Bed count: 100   Bassinet count: 15

Service	Live Adm.	Disch.	Deaths	IPSD	DD
Medical	166	163	10	859	845
Surgical	101	97	2	754	751
OB	92	93	1	365	369
Gynecology	81	80	1	313	325
Urology	60	57	0	231	240
NB	90	93	1	349	352

Calculate:

    a. Average length of stay.

    b. Average length of stay for each service:
       1) medical   4) gynecology

       2) surgical   5) urology

       3) obstetrics   6) newborn

c. * (R4) Occupancy percentage for October:

  1) bed

  2) bassinet

d. * (R5) Gross death rate for October.

12. Oceanside Hospital
   Clinical unit: Medical Service   Bed count: 50

Month	Adm.	Disch.	Deaths	IPSD	DD
Jan.	250	248	10	1250	1270
Feb.	223	231	8	1275	1266
Mar.	266	264	7	1266	1295
Apr.	245	251	5	1281	1254
May	248	244	4	1279	1287
June	212	213	4	1260	1310
July	218	217	6	1225	1263
Aug.	227	225	9	1248	1240
Sept.	259	260	7	1290	1233
Oct.	271	266	12	1313	1322
Nov.	275	272	10	1326	1333
Dec.	244	246	9	1288	1301
Totals	2938	2937	91	15,301	15,374

Calculate:

a. Average length of stay for the year.

b. Month with the shortest length of stay.

c. Month with the longest length of stay.

d. * (R4) Bed occupancy percentage for the year.

e. * (R4) Month with the best bed occupancy percentage.

f. * (R4) Month with the poorest bed occupancy percentage.

g. * (R5) Gross death rate for the year.

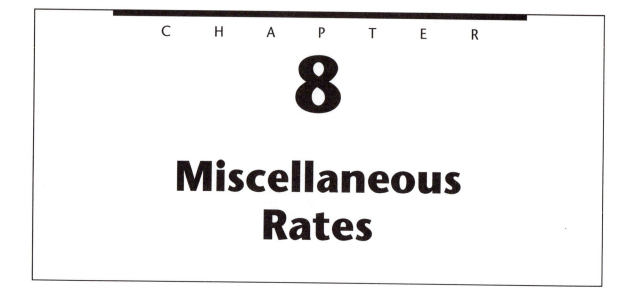

CHAPTER OUTLINE

A. Rates
   1. Cesarean Section Rate
   2. Consultation Rate
   3. Infection Rates

   4. Bed Turnover Rate
B. Summary
C. Chapter 8 Test

LEARNING OBJECTIVES

After studying this chapter the learner should be able to:

1. Distinguish clearly between
   a. Delivery vs. undelivered
   b. Birth vs. delivery
   c. Surgical procedure vs. surgical operation
2. Define "consultation."
3. Define "nosocomial infection."

4. Identify which infections are "postoperative infections."
5. Compute the following rates:
   a. C-Section
   b. Consultation
   c. Nosocomial infection
   d. Postoperative infection
   e. Bed/bassinet turnover

Other rates that are used by health care facilities are included in this section. The principle behind all these rates (and any others that your health care facility might devise) is based on the basic "rate formula" referred to in previous chapters—the ratio of the number of times something *does* happen compared to the number of patients to whom it *could* happen. Try to originate the formula for each of the rates in this chapter yourself, rather than looking immediately at the stated formula. With the increased availability and use of computers in health care facilities and the ability to collect and store data more efficiently, the probability of computing a wide array of rates and percentages is greatly increased. Facilities can now calculate anything from the rate of readmissions to the percentage of patients seen in consultation. Included in this text are rates that are calculated routinely in many health care facilities.

A. RATES

1. *Cesarean Section Rate*

Many hospitals determine the percentage of deliveries performed by C-section (Cesarean section) as compared to vaginal deliveries. Many hospitals have decreased the number of surgical deliveries. In some situations, their action could be the result of media coverage of the statistics related to surgical deliveries.

a. *Delivery*

The term delivery was defined in Chapter 5 when maternal death rates were discussed. It is important to remember that a delivery refers to expelling a product of conception or having it removed from the body. Multiple births constitute *one* delivery, although each infant delivered live is a newborn and each delivered without signs of life is a fetal death. Consequently, a woman who delivers quintuplets is credited with one delivery, just as a woman who gives birth to a single infant is credited with a single delivery. However, the number of births (newborn admissions) will be increased by five when live quintuplets are born, in contrast to an increase of one newborn when a single infant is born.

b. *Not Delivered*

This term includes pregnant females who were admitted to a hospital for a condition of pregnancy, but who did not deliver either a liveborn or stillborn infant during that hospitalization. This category includes threatened abortions and false labor, or treatment of a pregnancy-related condition.

c. *Cesarean Section Rate*

Formula:

$$\frac{\text{Total number of Cesarean sections performed in a period}}{\text{Total number of } \textit{deliveries} \text{ for the period}} \times 100$$

Example: A total of 220 deliveries are recorded by the obstetrical unit of a hospital. Of these 220 deliveries, 50 were performed by Cesarean section (C-section). In this instance, the Cesarean section rate is 50 divided by 220, and then the quotient is multiplied by 100, giving a rate of 22.7% [(50 ÷ 220) × 100].

Example: The obstetrical service lists 100 admissions for February. Discharges on the obstetrical unit total 103. Deliveries are reported as 77, and 22 were reported to be undelivered. Of the deliveries, 21 are accomplished by Cesarean section.

Twins were born to two mothers, and one mother gave birth to triplets. The only information needed is the number of Cesarean sections and the number of deliveries, irrespective of the number of infants delivered. Therefore, 21 C-sections occupy the numerator and 77 deliveries occupy the denominator. Dividing 21 by 77, and then multiplying the quotient by 100, results in a Cesarean section rate of 27.3% [(21 ÷ 77) × 100].

Note: Do not confuse newborn births with deliveries. A woman may give birth to either a live infant or a dead fetus, but each of the births would be considered a delivery. Also, a delivery may include more than one newborn, as was already mentioned.

SELF-TEST 36

Answers should be correct to *two* decimal places.

1. July obstetrical data:

OB admissions	451
OB discharges	456 (3 of which died)
Deliveries	446 (includes 4 sets of twins)
Undelivered	7
Cesarean sections	6

   Calculate: Cesarean section rate for July.

2. October obstetrical statistics:

OB admissions	65
OB discharges (live)	60
OB deaths	1
Undelivered	5

   Delivered:

		Total	Number Delivered by C-Section
Live:	Single infant	50	15
	Twins	3 sets	1 set
	Triplets	1 set	0
Dead:	Stillborn	1	1
	Aborted	1	0

   Calculate:

   a. Number of newborn births recorded in October.

   b. Total number of deliveries recorded in October.

   c. Number of newborn deaths recorded in October.

   d. C-section rate for October.

3. May OB statistics:

   OB admissions   78

   OB discharges (live)   72

   OB deaths   0

   Undelivered   4

   Delivered:

		Total	Delivered by C-Section	Deaths
Live:	Single infant	60	15	1 (at 36 hrs)
	Twins	4 sets	0	0
Dead:	Early fetal	3	0	
	Intermediate fetal	1	0	
	Late fetal	1	1	

   Calculate:

   a. Number of newborn admissions recorded in May.

   b. Number of newborn deaths recorded in May.

   c. Total deliveries recorded in May.

   d. C-section rate for May.

4. A hospital reports that there were 150 deliveries during October, fifteen of which were performed by C-section. Of the deliveries, 35 mothers were primiparous and five of these mothers were delivered by C-section.
   a. *Originate* a formula to find the percentage of women who delivered for the first time.

   Calculate:

   b. Percentage of mothers who delivered for the first time.

   c. A hospital needs to know the percentage of first-time mothers who had a C-section. *Originate* a formula to calculate this percentage.

   Calculate:

   d. Percentage of all C-sections that were performed on first-time mothers.

   e. Percentage of first-time mothers who had a C-section delivery.

2. Consultation Rate

A consultation has been defined as "a deliberation by two or more physicians with respect to the diagnosis or treatment in any particular case." A patient's attending physician sometimes requests a consultant to see his/her patient and offer an opinion, either to confirm a diagnosis or to treat a condition that is not in the attending physician's area of expertise. The consultant evaluates the patient and then must prepare a consultation report that includes the findings and recommendations for treating the patient's condition.

a. Consultation Rate

Formula:

$$\frac{\text{Total number of patients receiving consultation}}{\text{Total number of patients discharged}} \times 100$$

Example: A pediatric unit discharged 100 patients during the past month. Of these, 33 were seen by a consultant. Taking the number of consultations (33) and dividing by the total number of pediatric patients discharged (100), and then multiplying the quotient by 100, results in a rate of 33% [(33 ÷ 100) × 100].

SELF-TEST 37

1. During the first quarter of the year, it was reported that 2013 patients (1961 = A&C; 52 = NB) were seen in consultation by at least one consultant during their hospital stay. Of this number, 1008 (988 = A&C; 20 = NB) were seen by two or more consultants during their stay. A total of 3575 adults/children were admitted during this first quarter of the year, and 635 newborns were admitted. Discharges totaled 3568 for adults/children and 621 for newborns during the same period. Deaths recorded were 32 adults/children and two newborns. Inpatient service day totals were 20,331 for adults/children and 4052 for newborns.

   Calculate:

   a. Percentage of patients seen in consultation during their hospital stay during the first quarter of the year.

   b. Percentage of hospitalized patients seen by more than one consultant during their hospital stay during the first quarter of the year.

2. Glad Tidings Hospital reports the following statistics:

Service	Adm.	IPSD	Disch.	Deaths	Patients Seen in Consultation
Medical	998	15,203	991	18	312
Surgical	604	9,585	607	15	204
OB	378	4,219	372	2	85
NB	345	4,116	346	2	36
Psychiatric	207	3,028	202	3	44

   Calculate:

   a. Percentage of patients seen in consultation.

   b. Clinical service with the lowest percentage of patients seen in consultation.

   c. Clinical service with the highest percentage of patients seen in consultation.

3. A pediatric ward records the following statistics for May:

Bed count   12

Admissions   30

Discharges   28

Deaths   1   (under 48 hrs) (patient autopsied)

IP service days   300

Nosocomial infection   1

Seen in consultation   8   (6 were seen by two or more consultants)

Calculate:

a. Percentage of pediatric patients seen by a consultant in May.

b. Percentage of pediatric patients seen by two or more consultants in May.

c. * (R5) Pediatric death rate in May.

d. * (R6) Pediatric autopsy rate for May.

e. * (R4) Pediatric bed occupancy percentage for May.

3. Infection Rates (Morbidity Rates)

Hospitals try diligently to prevent hospital-borne infections from affecting their patients. Sterilized instruments are used, contaminated materials are appropriately discarded, and other measures are instituted to prevent the spread of infection. However, there is always the danger of acquiring a hospital-based infection, which is also called a nosocomial infection. (An infection that pertains to or originates in a hospital is a *nosocomial infection*.) Infection-control committees are charged with preventing and investigating nosocomial infections. All types of infections—such as respiratory, gastrointestinal, skin, urinary tract, surgical wound, septicemias, and those related to insertion of catheters—may be included.

Infection rates may include the entire hospital or be determined for a specific clinical unit (pediatrics, for example). Also, hospitals may choose to compute rates for various types of infection, such as urinary tract infections or respiratory tract infections. Ideally, the percentages will be low for nosocomial infections (morbidity rates). A health care facility should not have rates in the two-digit (more than 10%) range, and the computed rate may even fall below 1% (for instance, 0.5%). It is recommended that rates be rechecked (especially for decimal places) when a higher number than expected results.

a. *Hospital Infection Rate (Nosocomial Rate)*

Formula:

$$\frac{\text{Total number of infections}}{\text{Total number of discharges (including deaths)}} \times 100$$

Example: A total of 200 newborns were discharged during the past month. Twenty infants developed respiratory infections during their hospital stay. Placing 20 (the number of infants who developed an infection) in the numerator and dividing by the number of discharges (200), and then multiplying the quotient by 100, gives an infection rate of 10% [(20 ÷ 200) × 100].

SELF-TEST 38

1. During the year, Good Time Hospital reported 12 nosocomial infections. During this same period, there were 3015 adults and children admissions and 3021 adults and children discharges. Also included in the report were 457 newborn admissions and 453 newborn discharges. Total deaths reported were 44 (42 A&C and 2 NB). The inpatient service day total was 55,500 for adults and children and 9426 for newborns.

   Calculate: Hospital nosocomial infection rate for the year.

2. During the year, Goodfellow Hospital reported the following:

Service	Adm.	IPSD	Disch.	Deaths	Nosocomial Infections
Medical	364	10,555	361	14	4
Surgical	206	6,821	200	10	5
OB	62	2,485	64	2	1
NB	40	1,718	42	1	1
Orthopedic	88	3,002	85	7	3

   Calculate:

   a. Nosocomial infection rate for the year.

   b. Percentage of orthopedic patients who developed a nosocomial infection.

   c. Clinical service with the highest nosocomial infection rate.

   d. Clinical service with the lowest nosocomial infection rate.

b. *Postoperative Infection Rate*

   Another specific type of infection is one that occurs postoperatively. The surgical team takes great care to prevent a surgical patient from becoming infected as the result of a surgical operation. Copious amounts of antibiotics are often used for irrigation during an operation to prevent the onset of a postoperative infection. However, infections do occur and facilities often keep records of these infections. With the aid of these records, reported infections are investigated and an attempt is made to prevent recurrences. As with any infection, it is not always possible to determine the exact time when the infection was acquired. It is not always clear, for example, whether the patient entered with an infection or the infection was acquired or transmitted in the hospital.

1) *Terms*

   a) SURGICAL PROCEDURE

      Any single, separate, systematic manipulation upon or within the body that can be complete in itself, normally performed by a physician, dentist or other licensed practitioner, either with or without instruments, is considered a surgical procedure. Surgical procedures are done to restore disunited or deficient parts, to remove diseased or injured tissues, to extract foreign matter, to assist in obstetrical delivery, or to aid in diagnosis.

b) SURGICAL OPERATION

One or more surgical procedures performed at one time for one patient using a common approach or for a common purpose is a surgical operation.

Explanation: An operation may include more than one procedure, but the procedures would have to be related, or performed for the same common purpose. A salpingo-oophorectomy is considered to be one operation but also two procedures that can be carried out at the same time through the same surgical approach. A patient who had a tonsillectomy and then a hernia repair would, however, have had two operations with two procedures.

2) *Postoperative Infection Rate*

Formula:

$$\frac{\text{Number of infections in clean surgical cases for a period}}{\text{Number of surgical operations for the period}} \times 100$$

Example: A hospital that recorded 10 postoperative infections during the past month and performed a total of 250 surgical operations would have a postop infection rate of 4%. (Ten infections divided by 250, and then multiplied by 100, computes to 4%.)

SELF-TEST 39

1. Careful Hospital records the following data for the surgical unit for December:

Bed count	35	
Admissions	150	
Discharges	142	
Deaths:		
Total	4	(one died under 48 hrs)
Postoperative	2	(less than 10 days = 2; more than 10 days = 0)
Anesthesia	1	
Autopsies	3	
IP service days	943	
Patients operated on	138	
Surgical operations performed	164	
Anesthesia administered	168	
Patients seen in consultation	41	

Infections:

Nosocomial	2
Postoperative	4

Calculate:

a.   Postoperative infection rate for December.

b.   * (R5) Postoperative death rate for December.

c.   Nosocomial infection rate for surgical patients for December.

d.   Percentage of surgical patients seen in consultation in December.

e.   * (R4) Surgical unit bed occupancy percentage rate for December.

f.   * (R5) Anesthesia death rate for December.

2.   Surgical statistics for January:

Bed count	40	
Admissions	176	
Discharges	172	
Deaths:		
Total	5	(under 48 hrs = 2; over 48 hrs = 3)
Postoperative	2	(less than 10 days = 2; more than 10 days = 0)
Anesthesia	1	
Autopsies	4	
IP service days	1025	
Infections:		
Postoperative	3	
Nosocomial	2	
Patients seen in consultation	48	
Patients operated on	166	
Surgical operations performed	185	
Anesthesia administered	170	

Calculate:

a.   * (R5) Postoperative death rate for January.

b.   Postoperative infection rate for January.

c.   January nosocomial infection rate for surgical patients.

d.   Consultation rate for surgical patients for January.

e.   * (R5) Anesthesia death rate for January.

f.   * (R5) Gross death rate for surgical patients for January.

g.   * (R5) Net death rate for surgical patients for January.

h.   * (R4) Bed occupancy percentage for surgical patients for January.

3.   Surgical statistics for the first quarter (January through March):

Bed count   36
Admissions   360
Discharges   348
IP service days   2923
Patients seen in consultation   120

Additional Data:

Month	Deaths			Infections		Patients Operated on	Surg. Oper.	Anes. Admin.
	Anes.	Postop.	Other	Noso.	Postop.			
Jan.	1	1	1	1	1	108	120	110
Feb.	0	1	1	1	1	95	98	97
Mar.	0	2	0	1	2	123	133	125

Calculate:

a.   * (R5) Month (of the three-month period) in which the postoperative death rate was the highest.

b.   * (R5) Postoperative death rate for the period.

c.   * (R5) Anesthesia death rate for the period.

d.   Postoperative infection rate for the period.

e.   Month (of the three-month period) in which the postoperative infection rate was the highest.

f.   * (R4) Bed occupancy percentage for the period.

g.   Nosocomial infection rate for the period.

h.   * (R3) Average daily inpatient census for the period.

i.   * (R5) Gross death rate for the three-month period.

4. Surgical statistics for the week of June 1 through June 7:

Bed count: 40

Beginning census: 34

	6-1	6-2	6-3	6-4	6-5	6-6	6-7
Admissions	5	4	6	3	5	3	1
Discharges	3	5	2	4	6	4	7
Deaths:							
Total	0	0	0	1	0	1	0
Postop.				1			
Anes.						1	
IP service days	37	35	40	38	38	36	30
Infections:							
Postop.	0	0	1	0	0	0	0
Nosocom.	0	0	0	0	1	0	0
Patients operated on	2	7	5	6	3	8	2
Surgical operations	3	8	5	7	3	8	3
Anesthesia administered	2	7	6	6	4	8	3

Calculate:

a. * (R3) Census at midnight on June 7.

b. * (R3) Average daily inpatient census for the week.

c. * (R4) Bed occupancy percentage for the week.

d. * (R5) Gross death rate for the week.

e. Postoperative infection rate for the week.

f. * (R5) Postoperative death rate for the week.

g. * (R5) Anesthesia death rate for the week.

4. Bed Turnover Rate

Another measure of hospital utilization of beds is the bed turnover rate. This rate indicates the number of times each of the hospital's beds changed occupants.

Several formulae are in use for determining this rate and there is no universal agreement on the most accurate representation or formula. However, administrators of acute care hospitals are increasingly interested in bed turnover rates because they are considered a measure of bed utilization, especially in conjunction with percentage of occupancy and length of stay. When occupancy increases and length of stay decreases, or vice versa, the bed turnover rate makes it easier to see the net effect of these changes.

The following two formulae (which are among several that can be used) are used most frequently in the United States. They are referred to as the "direct formula" and the "indirect formula."

a. **Direct Bed Turnover Rate**

Formula:

$$\frac{\text{Total number of discharges (including deaths) for a period}}{\text{Average bed count during the period}}$$

b. **Indirect Bed Turnover Rate**

Formula:

$$\frac{\text{Occupancy rate} \times \text{number of days in a period}}{\text{Average length of stay}}$$

Example: A 200-bed hospital recorded the following during the past year.

Discharges: 7000

Average LOS: 8.5 days

Bed occupancy rate: 82%

Using the "direct formula," the bed turnover rate is 35 times. (7000 discharges divided by 200 beds = 35 turnovers.)

Using the "indirect formula," the bed turnover rate is 35.21. (0.82 occupancy rate × 365 days in a year divided by an average length of stay of 8.5 days = 35.21 turnovers.)

Therefore, during the year, each of the hospital's 200 beds changed occupants about 35 times.

c. **Bassinet Turnover Rate**

The same procedure can be followed to determine the bassinet turnover rate. Remember that A&C (adults and children) data and NB (newborn) data are generally kept separate with regard to census, percentage of occupancy, length of stay, and turnover rate.

d. **Usefulness of Turnover Rates**

Turnover rates can be useful in comparing:

1) One hospital with another.
2) Rates within the same hospital in terms of
    a) Utilization rate for different time periods.
    b) Utilization rate for different units.

For example, even though two time periods have the same percentage of occupancy, the turnover rates may differ. The rates may be lower because of a longer length of stay during one of these periods. If a unit has a high turnover rate—even though it has a low occupancy rate, such as might occur in the obstetric unit—this might be an indication of the greater number of patients being accommodated than in a unit (such as the surgical unit) with a higher percentage of occupancy but a longer length of stay. The bed turnover rate is generally regarded as a measure of the degree of bed utilization.

SELF TEST 40

Answers should be correct to *two* decimal places.

1. Shoreline Hospital reported the following during the past non-leap year:

	Beds	Bassinets
Count	250	15
Admissions	9205	1256
Discharges	9180	1245
Deaths	103	5
IPSD	69,608	4846
Discharge days	70,150	4888

Calculate:

a. * (R4) Percentage of bed occupancy for the year.

b. * (R7) Average A&C length of stay.

c. Bed turnover rate using the direct formula.

d. Bed turnover rate using the indirect formula.

e. * (R4) Percentage of bassinet occupancy for the year.

f. * (R7) Average NB length of stay.

g. Bassinet turnover rate using the direct formula.

h. Bassinet turnover rate using the indirect formula.

B. SUMMARY

1. Rates can be devised by dividing the number of times something happens by the number of times it could have happened.
2. A delivery involves giving birth—to either a living child or a dead fetus.
3. Multiple births constitute one delivery.
4. A surgical procedure is a single manipulation that can be complete in itself.
5. A surgical operation is one or more surgical procedures performed at one time using the same approach and for a common purpose.
6. Cesarean Section Rate: C-sections divided by deliveries.
7. Hospital Infection Rate: Infections divided by discharges.
8. Consultation Rate: Consultations divided by discharges.
9. Postoperative Infection Rate: Postoperative infections divided by the number of surgical operations.
10. Direct Turnover Rate: Discharges divided by bed count.
11. Indirect Turnover Rate: Occupancy rate times the days in a period divided by the average length of stay.

C. CHAPTER 8 TEST

Note: Answers should be correct to *two* decimal places.

1. Serendipity Hospital (July)

    OB Unit

Bed count	18	
Admissions	110	
Discharges (live)	101	
Deaths	1	(over 48 hrs)
Autopsies	1	(by hospital pathologist)
Delivered	89	(2 sets of twins)
Undelivered	12	
C-sections	27	

    Calculate:

    a. * (R5) Maternal death rate.

    b. * (R6) Maternal autopsy rate.

    c. C-section rate.

2. Cascade Hospital (August)

				Autopsies			Hospital
Unit	**Adm.**	**Disch.**	**Deaths**	**Yes (HP)**	**Coroner**	**Consults**	**Infections**
Medical	401	390	18	5	1	135	5
Surgical	88	81	2	1	0	61	2
Pediatrics	51	48	0	0	0	18	1
OB	268	269	0	0	0	12	2
GYN	47	45	0	0	0	3	0
Orthopedic	50	48	1	0	0	15	1
NB	241	239	1	0	0	2	2
Totals	1146	1120	22	6	1	246	13

    Calculate:

    a. Overall consult rate for August.

    b. Unit (service) with the highest consultation rate.

    c. Overall hospital infection rate for August.

    d. Unit (service) with the highest infection rate.

    e. * (R5) Gross death rate.

    f. * (R6) Gross autopsy rate.

3.   Windhaven Hospital (September)

Type of Surgery	Adm.	Disch.	Deaths	Patients Operated on	Consults	Postop. Infections
GI	36	35	1	34	12	1
GYN	45	44	0	43	3	0
C-section	21	22	0	20	1	0
Orthopedic	47	46	1	47	20	2
ENT	18	18	0	18	1	0
Urology	27	25	0	26	1	0
CV	22	20	2	20	10	1
Other	19	20	1	18	6	1
Totals	235	230	5	226	54	5

Other Statistics:

Surgical procedures   254

Surgical operations   235

Anesthesia administered   247

Calculate:

a.   Overall surgical consultation rate.

b.   Postoperative infection rate.

c.   * (R5) Surgical service with the highest death rate.

4.   Rainbow Hospital (June)

OB Unit		Deliveries		NB Deaths
		Vaginal	C-Section	
Admissions	283			
Discharges (live)	279			
Deaths	2			
Undelivered	21			
Delivered:				
Single	221	156	65	2
Twins	3 sets	2 sets	1 set	0
Triplets	1 set	1	0	0
Stillborn (all single):				
Early	17	17	0	
Int.	8	3	0	
Late	2	2	0	

Calculate:

a. Total number of live births.

b. Total number of deliveries.

c. Total number of newborn deaths.

d. C-section rate for June.

e. Percentage discharged undelivered.

5. Hillcrest Hospital (July)

				Autopsies					
Service	**Adm.**	**Disch.**	**Deaths**	**Yes (HP)**	**Coroner**	**Deliv.**	**C-Sect.**	**Infec.**	**Consult.**
Med	862	860	33	5	1			5	298
Surg	333	331	16	1	0			1	144
OB	257	255	1	0	0	237	66	2	8
NB	221	218	1	0	0			2	2
Totals	1673	1664	51	6	1	237	66	10	452

Calculate:

a. C-section rate.

b. Infection rate.

c. Consultation rate.

d. * (R5) Gross death rate.

e. * (R6) Net autopsy rate.

f. * (R5) Newborn death rate.

g. * (R5) Maternal death rate.

h. Surgical infection rate.

i. Medical consultation rate.

6. Riverview Hospital—OB Unit (June 10)

| Mother | Sex | Delivered via | | NB Weights | | Deaths |
		Vag.	C-Sect.	#1	#2	NB Maternal
J. Jones	M	*		8 lb 4 oz		
M. Myers	M		*	7 lb 9 oz		
S. Smith	F	*		6 lb 8 oz		
B. Brand	F	*		6 lb 11 oz		
D. Davis	M twins	*		5 lb 10 oz	6 lb 3 oz	
G. Grant	Abort M	*		450 gm		
C. Cooper	F	*		7 lb 3 oz		
L. Lyons	Abort F	*		950 gm		
N. Nolan	M		*	9 lb 1 oz		
P. Palmer	M	*		5 lb 1 oz		NB 10:55 A.M.
R. Rogers	F	*		8 lb 2 oz		
T. Turner	M		*	8 lb 9 oz		

Calculate:

a. Total number of newborn admissions.

b. Total number of newborn deaths.

c. Total number of deliveries.

d. C-section rate.

e. * (R5) Fetal death rate.

f. Percentage of live births who are male.

g. Average birth weight of liveborn males.

h. Average birth weight of liveborn females.

Exam—Chapters 3 through 8

Note: Assume that all questions on the exam relate to a non-leap year. Answers should be correct to *two* decimal places.

1. Beginning census   A&C = 180   NB = 10

Period	Months	Bed Count	Bassinet Count
A	Jan. through Apr.	200	30
B	Mar. through Aug.	220	30
C	Sept. through Dec.	210	30

Admissions:	A&C	NB
Period A	4036	648
Period B	4588	661
Period C	4271	653

Discharges:		
Period A	4025	645
Period B	4567	662
Period C	4272	650

			A&C		NB	
			<48 hrs	>48 hrs	<48 hrs	>48 hrs
Deaths:						
Period A	125	4	47	78	2	2
Period B	117	2	39	78	2	0
Period C	109	3	34	75	1	2

		Coroner				Coroner	
Autopsies:	*Path.*	*HP*	*Cor.*	*Path.*	*HP*	*Cor.*
Period A	51	4	8	2	0	1
Period B	42	3	7	1	0	0
Period C	34	6	4	2	0	1

ISPD:

Period A	20,227	1944
Period B	23,054	2015
Period C	21,475	1988

DD (Discharge days):

Period A	20,316	1977
Period B	23,129	2021
Period C	21,533	2004

Calculate:

a. Average daily inpatient census (DIPC) for each period and for the entire year for:
   1) A&C

   2) NB

b. Percentage of occupancy for each period and for the entire year for:
   1) A&C

   2) NB

c. Yearly death rates:
   1) Gross death rate

   2) Net death rate

   3) Newborn death rate

d. Autopsy rates for the year:
   1) Newborn autopsy rate

   2) Gross autopsy rate

   3) Net autopsy rate

e. Average length of stay (LOS) for:
   1) A&C

   2) NB

2. Lakewood Hospital (April)

   Bed count = 200
   Bassinet count = 35

	A&C	NB	OB	<10 days	>10 days
Admissions	1015	189	110		
Discharges	1002	181	104		

Deaths:

	A&C	NB	OB	<10 days	>10 days
Total	22	3	1		
Under 48 hrs	7	2			
Over 48 hrs	15	1			
Anesthesia	1				
Postoperative	7			3	4
Maternal 1					

	Deaths	Autopsies	
		HP	Cor.

Fetal:

	Deaths	HP	Cor.
Early	5	0	0
Intermediate	3	0	1
Late	2	1	0

Autopsies:

	A&C	NB
Pathologist	7	1
Coroner	2	1
IPSD	5286	816
Discharge days	5331	710

Infections:

	A&C	NB
Postoperative	1	0
Nosocomial	12	1
Consultations	316	15

OB: Delivered live:

Single	185
Twins	2 sets
Triplets	0

Delivered stillborn:

Single	10
Twins	0
Triplets	0
Undelivered	9

Type of delivery:

Vaginal	143
C-section	54

Anesthesia administered	331
Surgical operations	326
Patients operated on	318

Calculate:

a. Average daily inpatient census for:
   1) A&C

   2) NB

b. Percentage of occupancy for:
   1) A&C

   2) NB

c. Death rates:
   1) Gross death rate

   2) Net death rate

   3) Newborn death rate

   4) Postoperative death rate

   5) Anesthesia death rate

   6) Maternal death rate

   7) Fetal death rate

d. Autopsy rates:
   1) Newborn autopsy rate

   2) Fetal autopsy rate

   3) Gross autopsy rate

   4) Net autopsy rate

e. C-section rate.

f. Infection rates:
   1) Hospital infection rate

   2) Postoperative infection rate

g. Average length of stay for:
   1) A&C

   2) NB

3. Indicate whether or not each of the following is a *unit* of measure:
   a. Inpatient Service Day   Yes   No
   b. Inpatient Bed Count Day   Yes   No
   c. Inpatient Bed Occupancy Percentage   Yes   No
   d. Inpatient Bassinet Count Day   Yes   No
   e. Inpatient Census   Yes   No
   f. Average Daily Inpatient Census   Yes   No

4. An ice storm hits the local area. The hospital's 100 beds are filled to capacity and eight additional beds are set up in hallways and lounges and are occupied by patients. What is the bed complement for that day?

5. What is included in the numerator of death rates?

6. What is included in the denominator of autopsy rates?

7. What value occupies the numerator when the percentage of occupancy is being calculated?

8. What number is placed in the numerator when the average length of stay is being calculated?

9. Meadowland Hospital

Beginning Census	Period	Months	Bed Total	Med.	Surg.	OB	Bassinets NB
A&C = 123	A	Jan. through Mar.	130	65	40	25	20
NB = 18	B	Apr. through Sept.	145	70	45	30	25
	C	Oct. through Dec.	135	70	35	30	25

	Medical Unit				Surgical Unit			
	Adm.	Disch.	IPSD	DD	Adm.	Disch.	IPSD	DD
Jan. Feb. Mar.	994	989	5169	4956	495	491	3410	3430
Apr. May June	1161	1158	5889	5814	543	538	3814	3708
July Aug. Sept.	1154	1150	5996	5923	551	558	3779	3881
Oct.	355	356	1889	1797	146	144	978	1010
Nov.	321	319	1883	1666	151	149	1001	1101
Dec.	333	338	1897	1708	138	144	990	1055
Period total	1009	1013	5669	5171	435	437	2969	3166
Total for year	4318	4310	22,723	21,864	2024	2024	13,972	14,185

		Obstetrical Unit				*Neonatal Nursery*		
	Adm.	Disch.	IPSD	DD	Adm.	Disch.	IPSD	DD
Jan. Feb. Mar.	450	448	2189	1740	400	398	1710	1266
Apr. May June	491	492	2610	1781	431	433	2188	1382
July Aug. Sept.	487	485	2597	1846	440	438	2197	1495
Oct.	165	164	801	625	140	138	688	482
Nov.	171	169	792	654	138	140	691	497
Dec.	170	176	823	671	137	135	701	489
Period total	506	509	2416	1950	415	413	2080	1468
Total for year	1934	1934	9812	7317	1686	1682	8175	5611

A&C:	Date	Adm.	Disch.	IPSD	DD	Date	Adm.	Disch.	IPSD	DD
	Dec. 1	25	22	127	119	Dec. 17	21	24	127	124
	2	21	22	120	123	18	17	19	121	99
	3	28	26	128	137	19	19	20	123	105
	4	23	25	127	130	20	23	22	121	119
	5	29	27	130	141	21	19	20	115	104
	6	18	21	118	112	22	15	18	112	95
	7	22	20	124	105	23	9	29	117	146
	8	24	26	127	139	24	8	18	90	90
	9	29	25	131	130	25	5	4	84	25
	10	25	27	128	141	26	23	6	101	29
	11	21	22	124	117	27	21	10	118	51
	12	18	16	119	89	28	18	16	114	77
	13	20	24	126	129	29	21	24	115	120
	14	26	24	130	123	30	16	28	117	138
	15	24	23	129	121	31	26	25	116	124
	16	27	25	131	132	Total	641	658	3710	3434

Unit	Deaths Total	<48 hrs	>48 hrs	Post op. <10	Post op. >10	Anes.	Autopsies HP	Autopsies Cor.	Anes. Admin.	Patients Operated on	Surg. Oper.	Surg. Proc.
Medical	58	19	39				18	2				
Surgical:	22	7	15	16	6	1	5	1	1998	1881	1910	2111
Thorac.	(2)											
GI	(6)											
Ortho.	(4)											
GU	(3)											
Other	(7)											
OB	2	0	2				1	0				
NB	8	5	3				2	1				
Fetal:												
Early	35						0	1				
Inter.	18						3	2				
Late	12						2	1				

OB Deliveries	Total Live	Total Still	Vaginal Live	Vaginal Still	C-Section Live	C-Section Still
Single	1659	65	1327	57	332	8
Twins	12 sets		7 sets		5 sets	
Triplets	1 set		1 set			

Unit:	Infections Nosocomial	Postop.	Consultations
Medical	83		2007
Surgical (total):	105	110	1589
Thoracic	(18)	(12)	(389)
GI	(22)	(20)	(251)
Ortho.	(26)	(31)	(312)
GU	(20)	(25)	(288)
Other	(19)	(22)	(349)
OB	45	8	326
NB	21		228

Outpatients: Deaths = 138

Autopsies =38 by hospital pathologist; 11 coroner's cases

Calculate:

a. Average daily inpatient census for:

   1) Medical Unit for November

   2) Surgical Unit for the year

b. Average daily census for:

   1) Newborns for January through March

    2) A&C for the year

    3) Newborns for the year

  c. Bed/bassinet occupancy percentage for:
    1) Obstetrical Unit for April through September

    2) Bassinet percentage for October through December

    3) Bed percentage for A&C for the year

  d. The following death rates for the year:
    1) Net death rate

    2) Postoperative death rate

    3) Anesthesia death rate

    4) Maternal death rate

    5) Newborn death rate

    6) Fetal death rate

    7) Gross death rate

  e. The following autopsy rates for the year:
    1) Net autopsy rate

    2) Gross autopsy rate

    3) Hospital autopsy rate

    4) Newborn autopsy rate

    5) Fetal autopsy rate

  f. C-section rate for the year.

  g. Consultation rate for:
    1) Surgical Unit for the year

    2) Neonatal Unit for the year

  h. Infection rate for:
    1) Postoperative rate for the year

    2) Hospital rate for the year

    i.   Average length of stay for:

         1) Medical Unit patients for the year

         2) Newborns for the year

         3) Adults and children for the year

    j.   Periods (A, B, or C) with the highest percentage of occupancy for the Medical Unit.

    k.   Bed occupancy percentage for December 25 through December 31.

    l.   Bed occupancy percentage for December 24.

CHAPTER

9

Frequency Distribution

CHAPTER OUTLINE

A. Introduction
1. Ungrouped Frequency Distribution
2. Grouped Frequency Distribution
3. Purpose of a Grouped Frequency Distribution
4. Arranging Scores

B. Terms Related to a Frequency Distribution
1. Range
2. Class
3. Frequency
4. Cumulative Frequency

C. Creating a Frequency Distribution
1. Determine High and Low Scores
2. Arrange Scores in Descending or Ascending Order
3. Determine Range
4. Determine the Number of Class Intervals
5. Set Class/Score Limits
6. Rules for Subsequent Computations

D. Summary

E. Chapter 9 Test

LEARNING OBJECTIVES

After studying this chapter the learner should be able to:

1. Distinguish clearly between
   a. Ungrouped vs. grouped distribution.
   b. Frequency vs. cumulative frequency.
   c. Class limits vs. class boundaries vs. class size or width.

2. Construct a frequency distribution, either ungrouped or grouped.

3. Determine the following:
   a. Range
   b. Number of classes
   c. Frequency
   d. Cumulative frequency
   e. Class limits
   f. Class boundaries
   g. Class size/class width

A. INTRODUCTION

Data that are collected on a group of people are initially nothing more than a collection of numbers arranged haphazardly in a disorganized array. Often, when these data are organized and analyzed in a systematic fashion, they become meaningful and interpretations can be made based on the scores that are derived from them.

Suppose that a hospital has in its data bank the cholesterol values—recorded at the time of hospitalization—of all patients admitted with an admitting diagnosis of AMI (acute myocardial infarction) and that a physician would like to examine these data. It is quite likely that he would prefer to have the data displayed in an organized way, usually in the form of a frequency distribution.

1. Ungrouped Frequency Distribution

Previously it has been mentioned that an ungrouped distribution is

a. a listing of all scores as they are obtained; or
b. a listing of these same scores arranged from the highest to the lowest, or lowest to highest.

With a large number of scores, it becomes necessary to group and tally scores to facilitate analysis of the data and to put these data into a more concise form.

2. Grouped Frequency Distribution

Once scores are ranked, it becomes obvious that in many instances the same score is recorded by more than one individual. When scores are grouped, a frequency distribution becomes a grouped frequency distribution. However, according to some statistics texts, a grouped distribution must include a grouping of two or more *different* scores. For example, in this situation, scores of 80 and 81 are grouped together rather than just single scores (such as all scores of 80, for example).

Grouping data has become routine and simple with the aid of high-speed computers, and is even more easily achieved by using the sorting features in software packages that are available for use on a personal computer (PC).

Although the grouping process generally destroys much of the original detail of the data, it is often the most effective way to handle a large array of data and still obtain a clear "overall" picture of the obtained data and the vital relationship made evident by those data.

For example, people can vary greatly in height. A newborn is measured in inches, whereas a genetic giant may be well over seven feet tall. If every height was recorded in inches and measured to the nearest inch, the number of classes or categories could be great. Say, for example, that the shortest newborn was 10 inches in length and the tallest adult was measured at 90 inches, then the number of individual categories would be 80. Even a height distribution that eliminates children and includes only adults can have a range of 30 or more scores if the shortest adult is 48 inches and the tallest 78 inches. For this reason, *grouped data* are often used.

Whenever the range of scores is large—even when like scores are grouped together—it can be difficult to grasp the representation of the data. It is generally conceded that when the range of scores exceeds, say, 20 to 25, further consolidation of data may be desirable. This can be accomplished by grouping contiguous scores and combining their frequency. The resulting tabular arrangement is referred to as a *grouped frequency distribution*.

3. *Purpose of a Grouped Frequency Distribution*

The two main reasons for classifying data into a grouped frequency distribution are to

a. *Bring Order to Chaos*

Scores are listed according to size, which reduces the disorganization present in the original array of data.

b. *Condense Data to a More Readily Grouped Form*

By bringing like scores together and recording the total number of times each occurs, a more concise and useful distribution results.

4. *Arranging Scores*

Scores are generally listed from the highest score to the lowest in the distribution. Occasionally the reverse is correct, especially if a low score is better than a high score.

B. TERMS RELATED TO A FREQUENCY DISTRIBUTION

Several terms that are used when grouping scores for a grouped frequency distribution are:
1. Range
2. Class
    a. Class interval
    b. Class limits
    c. Class boundaries
    d. Class size/class width
3. Frequency
4. Cumulative frequency

For illustrative purposes, the following data will be referred to in describing terms related to a frequency distribution. The figures represent the birthweights (in grams) of infants born to mothers who smoked and to non-smoking mothers.

Non-smokers: 3515, 3420, 3175, 3586, 3232, 3884, 3856, 3941, 3232, 4055, 3459, 3998, 4048, 3769, 3688, 3456, 3815, 3422, 3916, 3361, 3661, 3962, 3557, 3191, 3164

Smokers: 2608, 2509, 3600, 1730, 3175, 3459, 3288, 2920, 3021, 2778, 2466, 3270

Comparison of Birthweights (in grams) of Infants born to Smokers vs. Non-Smokers
(f = frequency; cf = cumulative frequency)

	Nonsmokers	*f*	*Smokers*	*f*	*Total cf*
4050+	//	2			37
3900–4049	////	4			35
3750–3899	////	4			31
3600–3749	//	2	/	1	27
3450–3599	/////	5	/	1	24
3300–3449	///	3			18
3150–3299	/////	5	///	3	15
3000–3149			/	1	7

	Nonsmokers	f	Smokers	f	Total cf
2850–2999			/	1	6
2700–2849			/	1	5
2550–2699			/	1	4
2400–2549			/ /	2	3
2250–2399					1
2100–2249					1
1950–2099					1
1800–1949					1
1650–1799			/	1	1

1. Range

The range is the interval spanned by the data. It is computed by finding the difference between the largest score in the distribution and the smallest. If the scores span an interval in which the highest score recorded is 108 and the lowest is 18, the range becomes 90 (108 − 18 = 90). In the illustration above, the range is 2325 [high score (4055) minus the low score (1730) = 2325].

2. Class

A class is a category into which a score can be placed. It is a single score in a small distribution and a grouping of scores in a grouped distribution. When summarizing large masses of raw data, it often becomes advantageous to distribute the data into classes or categories and to determine the number of individuals or scores to include in each class. All data is then assigned and distributed within these classes, resulting in what is called a *frequency distribution*.

Example: If height measurements were made to the nearest inch, the heights could be divided into classes, thereby grouping together those within a range. One class could include all heights from 60 to 64 inches; the next class would then include heights from 65 to 69 inches; and so on.

Illustrative Example: Once the birthweights are arranged in order of size (from high to low), then categories or classes need to be assigned into which the scores can be grouped. Assuming that 150 consecutive scores (for example, birthweights of 1650 grams through 1799 grams) are all to be included in the same category, this category then comprises a class.

a. Class Interval

A class interval is a range of scores. An entire distribution is subdivided into intervals that contain all the scores within the range.

Example: A class interval with limits of 60 to 64 contains all the scores of 60, 61, 62, 63, and 64. Interval limits of 10 to 12 include the scores of 10, 11, 12. A distribution may also have limits of 80% to 89%, within which scores over 80% but less than 90% would be recorded.

Illustrative Example: All birthweights of 1650 grams through 1799 grams (up to 1800 grams) are included in the lowest interval of the distribution. The next class interval includes scores of 1800 grams up to, but not including, 1950 grams.

b. **Class Limits (Score Limits)**

The end numbers of the class interval are the class limits. The smaller number is the *lower class limit* and the larger number is the *upper class limit*. Class limits are also referred to as score limits or raw score limits.

Example: Referring to the example of heights, a class interval of 60 to 64 inches has a *lower* class limit of 60 and an *upper* class limit of 64.

Illustrative Example: The lowest class interval has a lower class limit of 1650 grams and an upper class limit of 1799 grams.

c. **Class Boundaries**

When measuring continuous variables with scores recorded to the "nearest whole number," the score is actually somewhere between 0.5 before the number or 0.5 following the number. For example, in recording heights to the nearest inch, an individual who is between 5 feet 5 1/2 inches and 5 feet 6 1/2 inches is recorded as 5 feet 6 inches in height. A class interval of 60 to 64 inches theoretically includes all measurements from 59.50 to 64.50 inches. This is the same principle on which *rounding* of numbers is based. These decimal numbers are the class boundaries. Again, the smaller number is the *lower* class boundary and the larger number the *upper* class boundary.

Class boundaries are also referred to as real or actual class limits, or true class limits.

Illustrative Example: Using the lowest class interval, the class boundaries are 1649.5 to 1799.5, which means that an infant needed to weigh at least 1649.5 grams, but not more than 1799.5 grams, to fall into this class interval.

d. **Class Size/Class Width**

The size or width of a class interval is the difference between the lower and upper class limit or class boundaries and is referred to as *class width, class size,* or *class length*. It is the number of scores grouped together in an interval, not the scores themselves. Traditionally, the interval size is the same for the entire distribution. However, in some distributions the class intervals will vary. To determine the size of a class interval of equal width, subtract two successive *lower* class or *upper* class limits.

Example: If heights are being recorded in inches and the interval limits have been set at 40–44, 45–49, 50–54, 55–59, and so on, then the class width is five [obtained by subtracting the lower limit (40) from the next lower limit (45), or subtracting two successive upper limits (49 – 44)].

Illustrative Example: The class width in the distribution is 150 scores—1800 (lower class limit of the second interval) minus 1650 (lower class limit of the lowest interval), which equals 150.

The size of the interval to be used is a matter of arbitrary choice; however, it is dependent upon several factors:

1) the nature of the data;
2) how this grouped distribution is to be used; or
3) the kind of interpretation that one desires to draw from it.

Generally speaking, the more detailed the interpretation one needs, the smaller the class interval size should be and,—as interval size increases—the more detail is lost. If high descriptive precision is needed or desired, if fluctuations in frequency over small parts of the range are to be studied, and if the number of scores tabulated is large enough to permit such detailed study, then the interval should be small. If, however, only a very rough picture of the distribution of scores is needed, a very broad interval may be quite satisfactory.

3. *Frequency*

Frequency refers to the number of times a certain score appears in the distribution. Frequency may be determined by counting the tally marks for each class or category. With the use of computers, frequency can be counted directly without having to first tally the scores.

Illustrative Example: The frequencies are recorded for each class interval for both smokers and non-smokers; the lowest class interval has a frequency of zero for non-smokers and one for smokers.

4. *Cumulative Frequency*

The cumulative frequency is the sum of the frequencies, starting at the lowest interval and including the frequencies within that interval. This column is prepared by "adding in" successive class frequencies from the bottom to the top. The entry opposite the lowest interval is the frequency in that interval; the entry opposite the second interval is the sum of the frequencies in the first and second intervals; the entry opposite the third interval is the sum of the frequencies in the first, second, and third intervals, and so on. The entry opposite the top interval would equal the total number of scores in the distribution. Cumulating frequencies is most commonly done from bottom to top, but it is also possible to cumulate from the top downward.

Steps to follow in cumulating frequencies:

a. *First Row*

Enter lowest frequency in cumulative frequency column of the first row (bottom row). In this first row, the frequency and cumulative frequency will have identical scores.

Illustrative Example: The only frequency (1) recorded was in the smokers column. This number is then placed in the adjacent cf (cumulative frequency) column (1).

b. *Second Row*

Add the frequency for the second row to the first row and record this total in the cumulative frequency column.

Illustrative Example: The frequency from the first row (1) is added to the frequency of the second row (0), resulting in a cumulative frequency of 1 (1 + 0 = 1).

c. *Subsequent Rows*

Continue adding the previous cumulative frequency to the next row's frequency, recording each total in the cumulative frequency column.

Illustrative Example: Refer to the distribution above and add the frequency in each row to the cumulative frequency in the previous row.

d. *Top Row*

The top row's cumulative frequency should equal N (the total number of scores in the distribution).

Illustrative Example: A total of 37 birthweights were recorded—25 were born to non-smokers and 12 were born to smokers. This total is called N, or the total number of scores. The cumulative frequency in the final row also is recorded as 37. These two numbers (N and final cf) should always be identical.

If you are cumulating from the top downward, then the final cf will be located in the bottom row of the distribution.

C. CREATING A FREQUENCY DISTRIBUTION

Steps to follow in creating a frequency distribution:

1. Determine High and Low Scores

Determine the highest score and the lowest score in the distribution.

2. Arrange Scores in Descending or Ascending Order (This Step Is Not Necessary but Is Extremely Helpful)

Beginning with the high score, list all scores from the highest to the lowest in the distribution. This convention should be followed unless some compelling reason dictates that the lowest score be placed at the top and the highest score at the bottom.

3. Determine Range

Subtract the lowest score from the highest score.

4. Determine the Number of Class Intervals

As a general rule, for most types of data, it is commonly recommended that the number of class intervals be at least 10 but no more than 20, with 15 classes being the preferred average. Some texts recommend no less than five and others state no less than 12, but the majority recommend a minimum of 10 classes. Most authors choose 20 as the maximum number of classes. Remember, however, that the number of recommended classes is only a rule of thumb and that the number must be based on the data and the interpretations that are to be drawn from this data.

Although grouped data can account for a grouping error, the error is generally regarded to be so small or negligible that it can be ignored, unless an interval size results in a very small number of classes, say, below 10. Although anywhere between 10 and 20 different class intervals for grouping scores is generally satisfactory, more precision can be attained with a minimum of 12 class intervals. As a single number, 15 class intervals seems to be a good compromise for an overall choice. Some data will require more class intervals, and other data can be condensed without being affected by grouping error. For more information regarding class interval size and number of class intervals, the reader is referred to a standard statistics text, which will include more details about these subjects.

5. Set Class/Score Limits

There is no universal rule governing how to set the limits of a class interval. Some common methods are included below, but it should be remembered that these are suggestions and that the limits should be representative of the data being grouped. Some statisticians recommend setting limits by beginning with the lowest interval, and others recommend starting at the top interval.

a. Suggested Methods

1) *Lower Limit a Multiple of Interval Size*

   A rather common method of setting the lower limit is to make the lower limit a multiple of the interval size. If the lowest score in a distribution is 19 and the interval size is determined to be three, the lower score limit of the first interval would be 18 and the upper score limit 20.

2) *Multiple of Highest Score the Middle Score of Interval*

   In this method a multiple of the highest score is found and this multiple should be the middle score of the interval. If the highest score is 178 and the interval size is three, the multiple computes to 177. In setting the score limits, the limits would read 176–178.

b. Departures from Convention

The practice of beginning a class interval as a multiple of class size or making the middle score of the uppermost interval a multiple of the highest score is a rule of thumb. There are instances when other limits are more applicable and the grouping is made easier. It is much easier to group large numbers of scores in multiples of 5 or 10. Score limits of 35–39 or 30–39 are much easier to work with than limits of 32–36 or 28–37. Therefore, limits are often set for the sake of convenience. Limits should be set by taking into account all the factors that will facilitate constructing the distribution and yet be representative of scores in the distribution. A little thought is required when setting class limits. However, in abandoning the rule, it is also possible that a bias can occur if the scores are not equally representative of the midpoint of the interval, because this midpoint is used in making computations from the grouped data. However, these errors will *not* be addressed in this text and the reader is referred to a more comprehensive statistics text for further analysis.

6. Rules for Subsequent Computations

For the sake of maintaining consistency among the computations that follow, the following rules will apply:

a. Desired number of class intervals—15, or between 12 and 20.

b. Preferred class sizes—1, 2, 3, 5, 7, 10, 15 (or any higher multiple of 5).

c. Setting lower limits: Determine the class size. If the class size is an

   1) *Odd* Number—Find a multiple of this number nearest to the lowest score in the distribution. This multiple should be the lowest score in the interval. Other limits will be determined automatically from this.

   2) *Even* Number—Find a multiple of this number and make the lower limit of each interval a multiple of this number.

Example: For illustrative purposes, a familiar example will be used—the results of the final test scores for 100 students at Studious State University. The recorded scores are as follows:

58	68	73	61	66	96	79	65	86	69	94	84	79
80	65	78	78	62	80	67	74	97	75	88	75	82
77	89	67	73	73	83	82	82	73	87	75	61	97
74	57	81	81	69	68	60	74	94	75	78	88	72
75	88	85	90	93	62	77	95	85	78	63	94	92
71	62	71	95	69	60	76	62	76	84	92	88	59
60	78	74	79	65	76	75	92	84	76	85	63	68
72	83	71	53	85	96	95	93	75				

a. Highest score = 97.
b. Lowest score = 53.
c. Range = 44. The lowest score (53) is subtracted from the highest score (97) for a range of 44 (97 − 53 = 44).
d. Class size = 3. The range (44) is divided by 15 (desired number of class intervals), which computes to a class size of 3.
e. Limits of the lowest class interval are 51 to 53. (The class size of 3 is odd and a multiple of this to the lowest score of 53 is 51. With a class size of 3 there will be three scores tabulated in the lowest class interval—51, 52, 53—resulting in limits of 51–53.)
f. Setting up the distribution:

Score Limits	Tally	Frequency	Cumulative Frequency
96–98	////	4	100
93–95	///// ///	8	96
90–92	////	4	88
87–89	///// /	6	84
84–86	///// ///	8	78
81–83	////// /	7	70
78–80	///// /////	10	63
75–77	///// ///// ///	13	53
72–74	///// /////	10	40
69–71	///// /	6	30
66–68	///// /	6	24
63–65	/////	5	18
60–62	///// ////	9	13
57–59	///	3	4
54–56		0	1
51–53	/	1	1

g. Number of classes = 16.

Example: If the scores in a distribution ranged from a high of 108 to a low of 18, the range would be 90. To find the number of intervals, the range is divided by 15 to approximate the number of scores that would need to be grouped into each class for a distribution of approximately 15 intervals. Dividing 90 by 15 results in a class size of 6 (90 divided by 15 = 6). However, 6 is not a preferred class size so 5 or 7 would more likely be used. Using 7 as the class size, the lower limit of the lowest class would be 14, a multiple of 7. The limits of this class interval would be 7–13. The resultant limits of the remaining classes are: 14–20; 21–27; 28–34; 35–41; 42–48; 49–55; 56–62; 63–69; 70–76; 77–83; 84–90; 91–97; 98–104; 105–111.

If the upper class had been established first by using a multiple of the highest score as being the middle score in the interval, then the top interval would read 102–108, because 105 is a multiple of 7 and becomes the middle score, with the remainder of the score limits following in succession as determined above.

SELF-TEST 41

1. For the scores below and, using the preferred class interval sizes, determine:
   a. The best class interval size for each range of scores.

   b. The approximate number of class intervals for these scores without setting score limits.

Score Limits	*a. Interval Size*	*b. Number of Class Intervals*
1) 1 through 45		
2) 72 through 136		
3) 43 through 237		
4) 0.12 through 0.38		

2. Determine approximately how many classes would result if:
   a. A class interval of 5 was used for a range from 1 through 55.

   b. A class interval of 5 was used for a range from 172 through 366.

   c. A class interval of 3 was used for a range from 88 through 124.

   d. A class interval of 10 was used for a range from 12 through 160.

3. Determine the range for the following high and low scores:
   a. 345 and 118

   b. 137 and 15

   c. 0.88 and 0.25

4. Indicate the class boundaries for the following class limits:
   a. 56 through 58

   b. 25% through 75%

   c. 0.28 through 0.30

5. For the following distribution, indicate the frequency for each interval and the cumulative frequency for each interval.

   Scores: 56, 51, 47, 58, 55, 52, 53, 52, 49, 55, 54, 53, 47, 51, 56, 57, 49, 50, 50, 48, 56, 58, 47, 57, 51, 54, 57, 49

Score Limits	Tally	Frequency	Cumulative Frequency
56–58			
53–55			
50–52			
47–49			

6. Set the score limits for the upper and lower intervals for a distribution in which 88 is the lowest score and 166 the highest.

D. SUMMARY

General Rules for Forming a Frequency Distribution:
1. Determine high score and low score.
2. Arrange scores in descending order.
3. Find range.
4. Determine the number of class intervals. Divide the range by 15 to approximate the number of scores to be grouped into each class for 15 intervals.
5. Set and list class interval limits for each interval. These limits should be set in ascending or descending order.
6. Tabulate and tally scores. Each data entry is tallied within each specific class interval.
7. Record frequency.
8. Check for accuracy. Total the numbers in the frequency column and make sure that total agrees with the total number of original scores, or compute the cumulative frequency as an accuracy check.

E. CHAPTER 9 TEST

1. The age of all patients is recorded when they are admitted to the hospital. The hospital administration would like a frequency distribution of the ages of patients who were admitted during the preceding year, excluding newborns. The oldest patient admitted was 102 and the youngest was a week-old infant. A total of 7823 patients were admitted during the preceding year.

   Determine:

   a. The size of a class interval.

   b. The number of class intervals.

   c. Score limits for each interval if zero is the lower limit of the lowest interval.

2. The ages of all cancer patients are recorded at the time the diagnosis of cancer is made. A total of 255 new cancer cases were reported during the past year. The tumor (cancer) registrar is asked to make a frequency distribution of this data. The youngest patient was three years old and the oldest was 92.

   Determine:

   a. Score limits for each class interval if the size of a class interval is five years and the lower limit of the lowest interval is zero.

   b. The number of class intervals.

3. A weight-reduction program for obese people was initiated for those who were at least 50 pounds over their ideal weight. A total of 86 people enrolled in the program at the beginning of the year and 45 of these 86 people remained in the program throughout the year. Their initial weights and final weights were recorded to the nearest pound, and the difference between these two weights was determined, resulting in the following data:

   –15, –26, –37, –55, –41, –18, –44, –9, –39, –22, 0, +5, –42, –33, –66, –24, –72, –33, –18, –29, –37, –43, –6, –46, –33, +10, –3, –51, –45, +12, –27, –53, –48, –19, –27, –46, –35, –62, 0, –18, –38, –28, –52, –16, –33

   Using an interval size of five, construct a frequency distribution, with the largest weight loss recorded at the top of the distribution and the weight gains at the bottom. Use the following headings:

   Weight Loss in Pounds   Tally   Frequency   Cumulative Frequency

   Hint: Lowest class interval limits are +10 to +14; +5 to +9; 0 to +4; –1 to –5; and so on.

4. A total of 320 patients was treated during the past year for STDs (sexually transmitted diseases). Excluding the 32 cases that resulted from congenital transmission or sexual abuse, construct the limits for a frequency distribution of the remaining cases (288) if the oldest patient was 88 and the youngest was 12.

5. Blood glucose levels are recorded for all males over the age of 40 who are admitted with a diagnosis of coronary artery heart disease. A total of 755 diagnosed cases were reported. The lowest blood glucose level recorded was 58 and the highest was 442. Using an interval size of 25, set the score limits for each interval.

6. Forty-eight patients were discharged during the past week. The number of clinical laboratory tests performed on each of these patients during their hospital stay was as follows:

   2, 15, 22, 31, 11, 18, 5, 7, 17, 3, 16, 1, 12, 9, 4, 6, 44, 7, 18, 4, 10, 14, 8, 13, 3, 3, 8, 11, 25, 29, 9, 21, 36, 2, 5, 6, 17, 8, 3, 9, 13, 9, 6, 5, 9, 14, 17, 12

   Construct a frequency distribution for these data, starting with an interval of 0 to 2.

7. A blood sample was taken from 100 smokers between the ages of 45 and 65, and then cholesterol levels were recorded. The cholesterol values were as follows:

199	240	255	181	178	181	287	219	218	256
267	209	199	382	246	234	179	286	273	296
166	171	240	288	198	257	289	224	221	225
239	255	198	175	249	186	243	194	235	274
189	232	192	277	231	211	241	298	230	248
251	238	147	211	196	202	231	240	216	187
223	268	201	239	213	189	185	195	234	290
279	231	203	259	230	164	212	217	238	199
190	199	243	163	134	219	205	186	214	228
235	221	266	244	199	263	301	284	217	223

   a. Determine the range.

   b. Determine the number of class intervals if 20 scores are to be grouped into each interval.

   c. Set the class limits for each interval if the lower limit of the lowest class interval is 130.

   d. Tabulate and tally the scores for each interval, and record the frequency and the cumulative frequency.

8. The blood pressures of patients discharged during the past month with a diagnosis of hypertension were reviewed. Eighty-four cases were found. Only the blood pressures recorded at the time of discharge were to be used in the study. The diastolic pressures (in mm Hg) were as follows:

88	98	78	84	77	81	90	82	75	72	100	92
85	92	77	84	77	82	92	88	74	80	95	90
87	80	83	77	86	80	88	90	79	82	93	88
80	85	96	85	90	84	82	95	88	97	105	80
94	92	88	96	90	88	86	84	90	98	102	88
86	95	97	88	75	82	90	98	84	97	100	84
78	80	82	86	90	85	95	88	86	90	101	88

   a. Determine the range.

   b. Determine the number of class intervals if the class size is two.

   c. Construct a frequency distribution with a class size of two, indicating the score limits, tallying the scores, and using a frequency column and a cumulative frequency column.

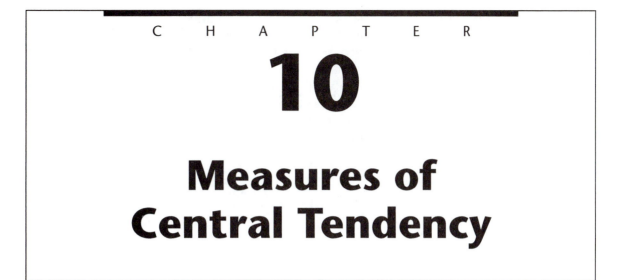

C H A P T E R

10

Measures of Central Tendency

CHAPTER OUTLINE

A. Mean
   1. Arithmetic Mean
   2. Weighted Mean
   3. Mean Computed from Grouped Data
B. Median
C. Mode
D. Curves of a Frequency Distribution
   1. Bilaterally Symmetrical Curves

   2. Skewed Curves
   3. Other Curves
E. Ranks/Quartiles/Deciles/Centiles/Percentiles
   1. Terms
   2. Percentages/Percentiles
F. Summary
G. Chapter 10 Test

LEARNING OBJECTIVES

After studying this chapter the learner should be able to:

1. Distinguish between the measures of central tendency—mean, median, and mode.
2. Distinguish between a bilaterally symmetrical curve and a skewed curve.
3. Distinguish between a curve skewed to the right vs. a curve skewed to the left.
4. Describe the effect of skewness on the measures of central tendency.
5. Distinguish clearly between a percentile rank and a percentile score.

6. Compare the advantages and weaknesses of percentiles.
7. Convert a score from a frequency distribution into a percentile.
8. Compute the following:
   a. Mean—arithmetic, weighted, from grouped data
   b. Median
   c. Mode
   d. Percentile from a grouped distribution

Measures of central tendency refer to scores that are most commonly called averages or values that are typical or representative of a set of data. Averages tend to lie near the center of a distribution when the data are arranged according to magnitude, and are therefore commonly referred to as *measures of central tendency*.

Several types of averages are commonly reported, of which the mean, median, and mode are referred to most often. If the frequency distribution is a bilaterally symmetrical, unimodal distribution, then all three measures of central tendency will be equal. Each of these measures has advantages and disadvantages, depending on the data and its intended purpose.

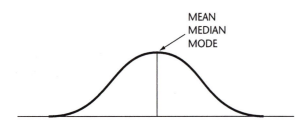

MEAN
MEDIAN
MODE

Relationship of measures of central tendency normal bell-shaped curve

A. MEAN

1. *Arithmetic Mean*

The mean (also known as the arithmetic mean) is an arithmetical average. It is computed in the same manner as an average (or averaging) is computed, as mentioned in Chapter 2.

Formula: Sum of All Scores (Σ) Divided by N (Total Number of Scores).

$$\frac{\Sigma \text{ scores}}{N}$$

Example: Seven patients were discharged from the hospital today and the number of days each was hospitalized was reported as 5, 3, 7, 12, 2, 4, 2 days, respectively. The average is the sum of the days (5 + 3 + 7 + 12 + 2 + 4 + 2 = 35) divided by the total number of patients (N = 7), for an average length of stay of 5 days.

SELF-TEST 42: Twenty-five patients were seen in the emergency room yesterday and the number of clinical laboratory and x-ray procedures performed on each patient was recorded as 5, 3, 7, 12, 18, 9, 10, 4, 20, 8, 15, 17, 22, 10, 5, 7, 21, 19, 15, 5, 9, 11, 8, 5, 5. Determine the arithmetic mean correct to the nearest whole number.

2. *Weighted Mean*

If certain scores (S) are more significant than others, they can be assigned a "weight" (W), depending on their importance.

Formula:

$$\frac{W(\Sigma S1) + W(\Sigma S2) \ldots; W(\Sigma S)}{W1 + W2, \ldots W}$$

Example: A final exam (FE) in a course is weighted three time (Q), and a regular exam (Ex) is weighted twice as much as a qu exams, five quizzes, and a final exam are administered during a cours mula for the weighted mean would be:

$$\frac{3\,FE + 2\,Ex1 + 2\,Ex2 + 2\,Ex3 + Q1 + Q2 + Q3 + Q4 + Q5}{3 + 2 + 2 + 2 + 1 + 1 + 1 + 1 + 1}$$

or

$$\frac{3(FE) + 2(Ex1 + Ex2 + Ex3) + 1(Q1 + Q2 + Q3 + Q4 + Q5)}{3(1) + 2(3) + 1(5)}$$

SELF-TEST 43: If the percentages for the tests in the previous example are FE = 85, Ex1 = 95, Ex2 = 90, Ex3 = 82, Q1 = 80, Q2 = 88, Q3 = 94, Q4 = 96, Q5 = 73, determine the average grade for the weighted mean correct to two decimal places.

3. Mean Computed from Grouped Data

When data are grouped into a frequency distribution, all the values that fall within a class interval are considered to coincide with the midpoint of the interval. In an interval whose limits are 60 to 62, all the scores within that interval would be considered to be 61 for computation purposes.

Example: A frequency distribution is made of the heights (in centimeters) of 100 males who are participating in a heart study:

Heights (cm)	Midpoint	Frequency	Freq. × Midpt.
175–179	177	2	354
170–174	172	12	2064
165–169	167	25	4175
160–164	162	32	5184
155–159	157	20	3140
150–154	152	9	1368
		100	

Total: 16,285

The mean is determined by dividing the total of all frequencies multiplied by their respective interval midpoints (16,285) by the total number (N) in the distribution (N = 100 in this distribution). The resultant mean or average height, in centimeters, of 100 male patients in the heart study is 162.85 cm (16,285 divided by 100).

SELF-TEST 44: A frequency distribution is constructed of the ages of patients at the time of death, as follows:

Age	Midpoint	Frequency	Freq. × Midpt.
90–104	97	4	
75–89	82	29	
60–74	67	25	
45–59	52	12	
30–44	37	7	
15–29	22	5	
0–14	7	8	

Determine: Mean age at the time of death for the above patients correct to the nearest whole number.

B. MEDIAN

The median is the middle score of a distribution when the scores are arranged in order of magnitude (from high to low, or low to high). It is the midpoint of a distribution, or the point above which 50% of the scores lie and below which the other 50% lie.

Formula: A. If N Is *Odd*—the Median Is the Middle Score.

B. If N Is *Even*—the Median Is the Average of the Two Middle Scores.

Example: Ten patients are seen for glaucoma screening. The intraocular pressures recorded are 14, 18, 20, 16, 24, 28, 10, 15, 21, 12. The scores arranged from high to low are 28, 24, 21, 20, 18, 16, 15, 14, 12, 10. Since ten is an even number, the median falls between the fifth and sixth scores, resulting in a median of 17 (18 + 16 = 34, divided by 2 = 17).

Example: The number of patients undergoing colonoscopy this past week were recorded as 2, 24, 18, 14, 17, 22, 28. The result of arranging the scores in order of magnitude would be 28, 24, 22, 18, 17, 14, 2. Therefore, the median is 18, because the middle score in a distribution of seven numbers is the value of the fourth score.

SELF-TEST 45: Fourteen new cases of cancer were reported during the previous week. At the time of their diagnosis, the ages of the patients were reported to be 18, 35, 50, 64, 88, 49, 75, 28, 61, 59, 47, 77, 66, 48.

Determine: Median correct to one decimal place.

C. MODE

The mode of a set of numbers is the score that occurs with the greatest frequency, that is, it is the most commonly occurring number (score) in the distribution. It is quite possible to have no mode in a distribution. Even if a mode does exist, it may not be unique. A distribution that has one mode is *unimodal*; a distribution that has two modes is *bimodal*. In a truly normal distribution, the mode score is found at the highpoint of the curve and is located in the center of that curve. It also will equal the median and mean in a normal, unimodal, symmetrical curve.

Example: Twenty cases of measles were reported during the past month. The ages of the patients are 12, 14, 18, 17, 20, 21, 9, 19, 22, 20, 19, 16, 21, 23, 21, 18, 10, 20, 21, 19. Since the mode is the score that occurs most often, the mode is 21 (four cases being reported in this age group).

SELF-TEST 46: Prior to the start of class, resting heart rates were recorded for all females who had signed up for a low-impact aerobics program. The rates for the fifteen females, ages 20 to 25, were 73, 77, 80, 83, 73, 82, 75, 73, 77, 84, 76, 81, 75, 79, 70.

Determine:

    a. Mode.

    b. Median.

    c. Mean, correct to the nearest whole number.

D. CURVES OF A FREQUENCY DISTRIBUTION

1. Bilaterally Symmetrical Curves

A curve that is bilaterally symmetrical is one that, when folded down the center vertically, is identical on both sides of the fold. In a bilaterally symmetrical curve, all three measures of central tendency (mean, median, mode) will be identical. These three measures will lie at the center of the distribution and thus they are called measures of central tendency.

a. Bell-shaped Curve

A bell-shaped curve is generally considered the mathematical ideal. It is a curve with a certain proportion and in which a certain percentage of scores lie at certain intervals along the curve. A bell-shaped curve is also referred to as a "normal curve."

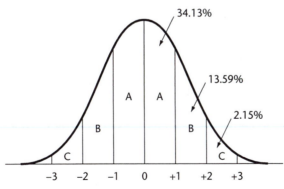

Normal bell-shaped curve

b. Other Symmetrical Curves

These curves resemble the bell-shaped curve and are symmetrical, but they vary in their ratios of height to width. Some are referred to as "peaked" curves and others as "flat" curves.

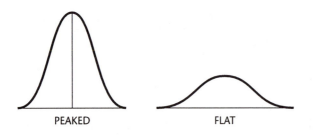

Symmetrical curves

2. *Skewed Curves*

Not all curves are symmetrical in shape. Those that have numbers piled up at the high or low end of the curve are called skewed curves. The direction of skewness refers to the location of the tail rather than to the side on which the piling up of scores occurs.

Skewness also affects the location of the measures of central tendency. Instead of all three measures being representative and identical, the location of each shifts. A curve skewed to the right has its mean shifted to the right (a higher number) and a curve skewed to the left will have its mean shifted to the left.

a. *Skewed to the Right (Positive Skewness)*

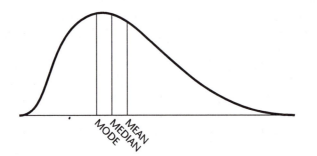

b. *Skewed to the Left (Negative Skewness)*

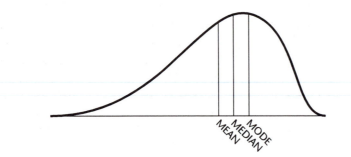

Example: The most common example of skewness in hospital statistics occurs when reporting and plotting the lengths of stay of inpatients when one or more of these patients has an exceptionally long stay—possibly a stay of over one year. This would result in a positive skewness (skewed to the right), thus raising the mean for all patients. To illustrate, the following discharges could be reported on a certain date:

Patient	Admitted	Discharged	LOS
Anderson, A.	3-03-89	3-10-89	7
Barker, B.	2-15-89	3-10-89	23
Carlson, C.	3-01-89	3-10-89	9
Daniels, D.	3-07-89	3-10-89	3
Edwards, E.	12-27-88	3-10-89	73
Foster, F.	3-05-89	3-10-89	5
Grant, G.	2-28-89	3-10-89	10
Hughes, H.	3-04-89	3-10-89	6
Ingold, I.	2-26-89	3-10-89	12
Jansen, J.	1-03-88	3-10-89	<u>431</u>
		Total:	578

Mean: 57.8 days (578/10)

Median: 9.5 days (The ten lengths of stay arranged according to magnitude are 431, 73, 23, 12, 10, 9, 7, 6, 4, 3. The middle score is found by computing the average of 10 + 9, or 9.5 days).

c. *Effect of Skewness on Measures of Central Tendency*

From the illustration above, it is obvious that extreme scores can greatly affect the mean of a distribution. However, it must be pointed out that average lengths of stay are usually computed on more than ten patients. The small number was included here for illustrative purposes only. It was used to show the influence of a nonrepresentative score on the mean of a distribution and the effect that one or more extreme scores can have on measures of central tendency, especially in skewed distributions. The reader should also be made aware that statistics must be taken with a "grain of salt" and that careful judgments must be made when reading or interpreting data.

d. *Reporting Measures of Central Tendency from a Skewed Distribution*

The term "average" is synonymous with the arithmetic mean but is often used to indicate either the mean or median. (The mode is seldom used as a representative measure of central tendency). The mean is not always the best indicator of what the data represents with regard to central tendency. If data are symmetrically distributed, either the mean or the median will be representative of the data. For a series with a large amount of data, the mean is easier to compute, whereas for a small series the median is more easily determined. Median determination is generally very time-consuming, unless a computer is used to more easily sort the data into a sequence by magnitude.

When the series is skewed, the median is the more representative measure of central tendency. As was pointed out in the previous section, even a few cases of extended stays can have a major effect on the computation of the mean. Therefore, the median is normally the average of choice for these types of data. When reporting data from a skewed distribution, it is generally advisable to attach a notation as to why the median was used rather than the mean, or to explain the reason for the higher-than-normal mean.

e. **Suggestions for Reporting Averages**

If a patient or a group of patients falls at the extremes of a distribution, there are several options to choose from in reporting averages.

1) *Calculate Mean and Attach a Notation to the Report*

   a) INCLUDE THESE PATIENTS IN THE CALCULATION

   If the distribution is skewed and the mean is computed, a statement of explanation should accompany the report—for instance, that one patient had a length of stay of over one year.

   b) EXCLUDE THESE PATIENTS IN THE CALCULATION

   Do not include the patient who severely skews the distribution, but include a statement of explanation for the exclusion—for example, that one patient had a length of stay of 400 days and was excluded in the computation of the mean.

   c) CALCULATE BOTH WAYS

   Include and *exclude* these patients. Calculate the mean both by including and excluding the patient in the computation, and attach a note to explain the difference in the two means.

   Example: If one patient stayed 431 days (over a year), a report might state that the average (mean) length of stay for all patients was 44.8 days, but that one patient had a length of stay of 431 days. By excluding that patient, the mean length of stay for all patients was 6.7 days.

2) *Calculate Median and Attach a Notation to the Report*

   Explain in the notation that one patient had an extended stay of 431 days and, for that reason, the median was chosen as most representative of the average length of stay of the hospitalized patients.

f. **Additional Points**

The median is the more representative measure of central tendency when a distribution is skewed. The few extremes in the tail of a distribution do affect the mean more than the median. It should be pointed out that this applies primarily to the acute-care hospital and not to extended-care sections of a hospital, because the lengths of stay of these patients would routinely be longer. When a small number of patients have exceptionally long lengths of stay, the true representative average of the majority of patients is distorted.

The major disadvantage of calculating the median is that it can be time-consuming. Manually arranging numbers in numerical order, especially a large number of them, takes far too long to be practical. However, since most hospitals are equipped with computers, this task becomes easily achievable by using the sorting and calculating capabilities of the computer. Remember that a notation explaining the effect or use of a measure of central tendency should accompany the report.

3. **Other Curves**

Shown on the following page are other types of curves that may be encountered in graphical representations of data. They are included here for reference purposes only.

a. J-shaped

b. Reverse J-shaped

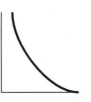

c. U-shaped

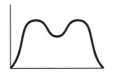

d. Bimodal

e. Multimodal

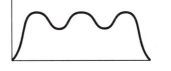

E. RANKS/QUARTILES/DECILES/CENTILES/PERCENTILES

It is not at all uncommon for an individual to be ranked in relation to other members of a group. Everyone has at one time or another been told that they ranked, for example, tenth out of 30 participants who took an exam or ran in a race, and so on. Most people are also familiar with a percentile ranking, such as placing in the top 10% of a class or group (or in the lower 10%).

1. TERMS

a. Rank

Rank indicates relative status in a group. The rank of a score indicates its position in a series when all scores have been arranged in order of magnitude. A rank of 30, for example, indicates that the score is 30th from the top (or from the bottom) when all scores have been arranged in order of magnitude.

The meaningfulness of any designated rank depends upon the number of scores in the series or distribution. To rank 30th in a group of 50 is not the same as ranking 30th in a group of 100 or 30th in a group of 30. For this reason, ranks are more appropriately expressed in more relative terms as percentiles.

b. Quartiles

Data arranged in magnitude can be divided into subparts. The median divides the distribution into two equal parts. By extending this concept, the distribution could be broken into four equal parts. Each of these four parts is called a quartile—the first quartile extends to the 1/4 mark, the second quartile to the 1/2 point (median or middle), and the third quartile extends to the 3/4 point of the distribution.

There are three quartiles—25th, 50th, and 75th. The 50th quartile is also the median of the distribution.

c. Deciles

Similarly, the data set can be divided into ten equal parts called deciles. The first decile includes 1/10 or 10% of the data in the distribution; the second decile another tenth (to the 20% mark); and so on. The fifth decile corresponds to the second quartile, or median.

There are ten deciles: 10th, 20th, 30th, 40th, 50th, 60th, 70th, 80th, 90th, 100th. The 50th decile is the 50th quartile and the median of the distribution.

d. Centiles/Percentiles

Percentiles divide the distribution into 100 equal segments. The first decile is the 10th percentile; the first quartile is the 25th percentile, etc. Percentile rank of a given score in a distribution is the percentage of measures in the whole distribution that are lower than the given score. When a person scores at the 90th percentile, it indicates that the score exceeds 90% of all scores of a set of observations and is exceeded by only 10%. The 50th percentile is the median of the distribution.

e. Percentile Rank

The percentile rank is the percentile for a specific score. For example, someone who scores a 67 on a test may rank at the 90th percentile. However, a score of 15 on another test may also be ranked at the 90th percentile.

f. Percentile Score

The percentile score is the score that one had to attain to reach a specific percentile. For example, to rank at the 90th percentile, an individual may have needed a score of 67.

2. Percentages/Percentiles

a. Importance of Percentiles

A raw score reported as 43 may not be meaningful to the person who achieved it. If, in addition, the person was told that this score placed him/her at the 85th percentile and that out of all those who took the test only 15% got a higher score, the person would have a better understanding as to his/her test performance in relationship to the entire group.

Example: A group of arthritic patients is undergoing daily range-of-motion exercises in the physical therapy department. One test involves standing upright and bending forward, in an attempt to touch the toes. Scores are recorded to the nearest half-inch, and are based on how close the fingers come to touching the floor. If 60% get to within two inches of the floor, any person who attains this level of achievement has a better indication of how he/she did compared to others in the group.

b. *Weakness of Percentiles*

Percentile scores are not equally divided up and down a percentile scale. If ten score points separate the 70th and 80th percentile, this does *not* mean that ten score points separate each decile level, because scores often tend to be clustered near the middle, with less of a spread within this range. Special statistical treatment is required to figure specific scores from a percentile score.

In percentiles:

1) The number of scores between each percentile is equal.
2) The score ranges between percentiles may be unequal.

c. *Cumulative Frequency Related to Percentiles*

The calculation of a cumulative frequency was discussed in the chapter on frequency distributions. It is computed in the same manner here—by adding each frequency to the previous frequency and accumulating frequencies with each row. Each row should be a total of all the frequencies up to that row. Remember that it is most common to cumulate from the bottom to the top, but it is also possible to cumulate from the top downward.

d. *Conversion of Cumulative Frequency into Percentage/Percentile*

An approximation of a percentile for a given score can be obtained quite easily by using a hand calculator. This approximation will be within a point or two of the true percentile.

Formula:

$$\frac{\text{Cumulative Frequency}}{N + 1} \times 100 = \text{Percentile}$$

If several scores are identical, they will have the same cumulative frequency and the cumulative frequency will need to be reduced by averaging the cumulative frequency for that score with the one below.

Example: A distribution has a single score whose cumulative frequency is 25. There are 80 scores in the distribution. To determine the percentile rank, the cumulative frequency of 25 is placed in the numerator and 81 (80 + 1) is placed in the denominator. The quotient is then multiplied by 100 for a percentile rank of 31 (30.86 is rounded to 31).

Example: Three scores are identical in a distribution and the cumulative frequency is 26. These three scores actually would have had cumulative frequencies of 24, 25, and 26 had they all been different. Taking the average of the three cumulative frequencies yields a cumulative frequency of 25. If there were 86 scores in the distribution, the percentile rank of these three scores would be 29 (25 divided by 86 + 1, or 87 and multiplied by 100, which computes to 28.74, which rounds to 29).

If two scores were identical and they had a cumulative frequency of 26, the two cumulative frequencies of 25 and 26 would be averaged and a cumulative frequency of 25.5 would be used in computing the percentile rank.

F. SUMMARY

1. Averages tend to lie near the center of a distribution and are commonly referred to as measures of central tendency. The mean, median, and mode are types of averages.
   a. Mean
      1) The arithmetic mean is the arithmetic average of the distribution.
      2) A weighted mean is used if certain components are more important than others.
      3) To compute the mean of grouped data, the midpoint of the score limits of each interval is used.
   b. The median is the middle score of a distribution when scores are arranged in order of magnitude.
   c. The mode is the most frequently occurring score.
2. A frequency distribution can be plotted as a curve. Curves may be symmetrical or skewed. The bell-shaped curve is also called a normal curve. Skewed curves are either skewed to the right or left (also referred to as positively or negatively skewed).
3. Skewed distributions affect measures of central tendency. The median is more representative of scores in a skewed distribution than is the mean.
4. A rank indicates relative status within a group.
5. Quartiles, deciles, and percentiles divide a distribution into subparts.
6. The percentile rank and percentile scores are identical.
7. Percentiles and percentages have strengths and weaknesses that should be considered before percentiles and percentages are used.
8. Percentiles can be determined from a grouped or ungrouped frequency distribution.

G. CHAPTER 10 TEST

Note: Where computations are called for, answers should be correct to *two* decimal places.

1. Given the series: 85, 87, 90, 94, 96, 97, 97, 98, 99

   Determine:

   a. Median.

   b. Mean to the nearest whole number.

   c. Mode.

2. An index is to be computed using the following weights: resting diastolic pressure, 3; resting heart rate, 2; serum cholesterol, 1. Readings are taken weekly for six weeks and then averaged for the period. A patient's average readings are as follows: diastolic pressure, 82; heart rate, 62; cholesterol, 164. What is the weighted mean?

3. Which measure of central tendency is largest if a frequency distribution is skewed to the right?

4. Which measure of central tendency is most representative of the scores in the distribution if the distribution is skewed?

5. The lengths of stay are recorded for patients admitted with coded diagnoses for poisoning or injury. They are as follows:

13	11	3	12	2	10	17	24	20	1	35	5	5	3	31
30	39	1	2	6	1	1	10	2	21	11	5	3	1	2
17	6	8	5	1	2	4	4	6	19	2	5	34	2	4
2	6	9	61	40	26	21	14	8	4	13	17	51	15	56
6	2	33	14	3	40	24	3	5	8	18	5	31	8	21
14	5	26	10	6	57	51	2	22	8	6				

Determine:

a. Value of N.

b. Mean from ungrouped data.

c. Median from ungrouped data.

d. Mode from ungrouped data.

e. Mean, using a grouped distribution beginning with a lower interval of 1 to 4.

f. Length of stay score at the
　1) first quartile.

　2) third quartile.

　3) 90th percentile.

　4) sixth decile.

　5) second decile.

g. Percentile rank of a length of stay of
　1) 33

　2) 18

　3) 9

h. Percentage of scores that fall below a length of stay of 12 days.

i. Percentage of scores that fall between one through four days.

j. Approximation of percentile rank for a length of stay of 22 days.

6. State the end (either right or left) at which scores tend to pile up with a

   a. positively skewed distribution.

   b. distribution skewed to the right.

7. Indicate the respective location for the mean, median, and mode for a negatively skewed distribution.

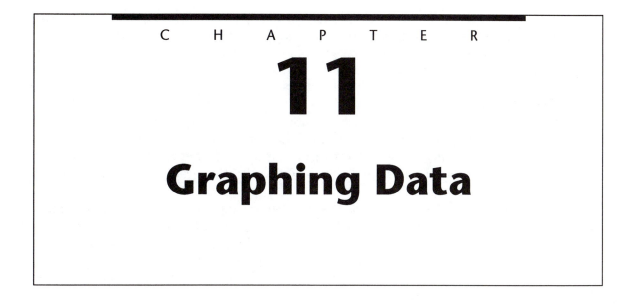

CHAPTER 11

Graphing Data

CHAPTER OUTLINE

A. Plotting a Frequency Distribution
   1. Axes
   2. Vertical Scale
   3. Scale Proportion
B. Types of Graphs/Charts/Diagrams
   1. Histogram
   2. Frequency Polygon
   3. Histogram and Frequency Polygon—
      Additional Information

   4. Bar Graph/Bar Chart
   5. Line Graph
   6. Pie Graph/Pie Chart
   7. Pictograph/Pictogram
   8. Comparison Graph
C. Summary
D. Chapter 11 Test

LEARNING OBJECTIVES

After studying this chapter the learner should be able to:

1. Indicate the appropriate types of graphs that can be used for displaying quantitative and qualitative data.
2. Distinguish the type of data presentation that is appropriate for different situations.
3. Construct the following:
   a. Histogram
   b. Frequency polygon

   c. Bar graph/Bar chart
   d. Line graph
   e. Pie graph
   f. Pictograph/Pictogram
   g. Comparison graph—both bar graph and line graph.
4. Distinguish among and interpret various kinds of graphs.

A graph is a pictorial presentation of the relationship between variables. Graphs are designed to help the reader grasp information more quickly and obtain a general picture of the data at a glance. An effective graph is simple and clean. A graph should *not* attempt to present so much information that it becomes confusing to the user and is difficult for the user to comprehend. An effective graph helps the reader obtain a quick overall grasp of the material being presented.

Many types of graphs are employed in statistics, depending upon the nature of the data involved and the purpose for which the graph is intended. Graphs are sometimes referred to as *charts* or *diagrams*. Thus, a bar graph is also referred to as a bar chart; a pie graph may be called a pie chart or pie diagram. Representative graphs will be included in this chapter.

Pictorial and graphic presentation of data is presently being used much more routinely because of the availability of software graphics packages, which are designed even for personal computers. No longer do most graphs, charts, or diagrams need to be plotted by the pen-and-ink method: the information can now be fed directly into the PC, which can then print out a very professional-looking graph or chart in a fraction of the time that used to be required by conventional means.

Color can also be an enhancement, helping to convey the meaning of the material being presented. When color is used, it is necessary to include a key to explain the representation. Shading and other means of highlighting can also be used effectively, as long as they are differentiated by means of a key that is included with the graph.

The major advantages of graphics are that they condense data into a form more readily grasped and that they facilitate the comprehension of trends that otherwise might be more obscure and uninterpretable.

A. PLOTTING A FREQUENCY DISTRIBUTION

The frequency distribution was introduced in Chapter 9 and individual scores were grouped and consolidated into a what is referred to as a "frequency distribution." This same data can be represented in graphic form. Included here are some rules to facilitate the plotting of such a distribution.

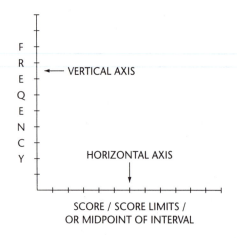

Plotting a frequency distribution

1. Axes

Most graphs have two axes—a *horizontal* axis and a *vertical* axis. As a general rule, when plotting a frequency distribution, one axis represents the score (or class interval) and the other axis the frequency. In the majority of cases,

a. the *horizontal* axis represents the score, score limits, or midpoints of the interval.
b. the *vertical* axis represents the frequency.

2. Vertical Scale

The vertical scale, as mentioned, indicates the frequency of the scores. The scale should begin at zero to avoid misleading the reader. If the data lends itself to a different lower frequency (other than zero), a broken line or other means of interruption should be drawn at the bottom of the vertical axis. This broken line should be employed as well at the bottom of each frequency rectangle to indicate clearly that the "zero frequency" rule was circumvented.

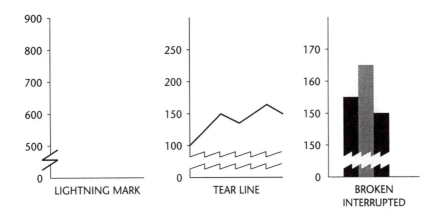

3. Scale Proportion

The scale of a graph or chart refers to the proportion or distribution of the two axes—the height and width of these axes in relationship to one another. As a general rule, the *height* of the vertical axis should be approximately 3/5 (60%) or 3/4 (75%) the *length* of the horizontal axis.

A graph in which the height exceeds the horizontal length, or otherwise deviates markedly from this proportion, may appear out of proportion with reality. If the graph is being constructed manually, graph paper facilitates plotting and saves construction time. Graphs can be enlarged or reduced on a copying machine to accommodate their intended use, whether within a text or as a visual display.

B. TYPES OF GRAPHS/CHARTS/DIAGRAMS

There are various types of graphic representation. Included in this section are some of the more common forms of presenting data in a graphic form.

1. Histogram

A histogram is probably the most common and simplest of the various graphic forms. A histogram is a pictorial or graphic representation of a frequency distribution or table, in which each frequency is shown by the height of a rectangle erected for each score. The rectangles designate the frequency for each score or class interval in the distribution.

A true histogram presents *quantitative* data (continuous data), never qualitative data. The horizontal axis is composed of the class boundaries rather than the score limits. The vertical axis depicts the frequency (designated on the frequency distribution). Rectangles are drawn for each class interval and are laid side-by-side, contiguous to each other, with *no* space between rectangles.

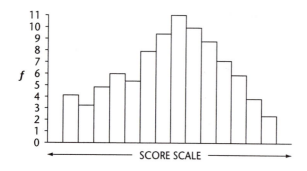

Histogram

a. Construction of a Histogram

1) *Lay Out the Horizontal and Vertical Axes*

2) *Mark the Axes*

   Indicate the marks on the vertical axis and the class boundaries along the horizontal axis.

3) *Draw the Rectangles*

   Draw a rectangle for each interval of the frequency distribution. Two vertical lines are constructed above each class boundary equal to the height of the class frequency for that interval (see line "a" in diagram below) and a horizontal line or bar ("b" in diagram below) is constructed along the top of each class interval, joining the two vertical lines to form a rectangle.

   Continue drawing a rectangle for each additional class interval in the distribution until all intervals are represented and the histogram is complete.

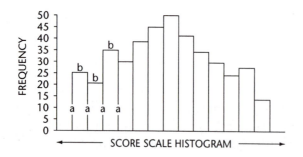

4) *Label the Axes*

Indicate what the data on each axis represents.

5) *Title the Histogram*

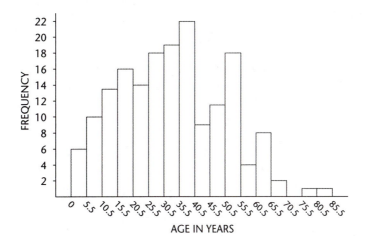

Traumatic hyphema diagnoses ABC Clinic (March 1994)

The area under each rectangle also corresponds to the percentage of total scores. To get a proper representation of data, it is imperative that the size of class intervals be identical. A histogram will be distorted if unequal class interval sizes are used and this distortion must be taken into account when constructing a histogram with unequal class intervals.

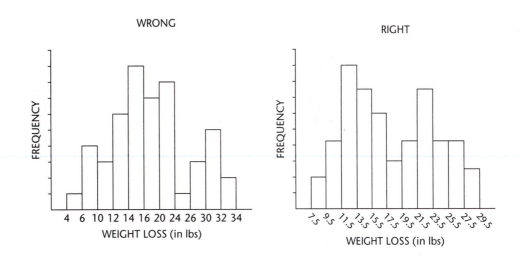

b. **Summary for Constructing a Histogram**

1) The vertical scale should begin at zero.

2) Use correct proportion between the scales—the height of the vertical axis should be approximately 3/5 or 3/4 the length of the horizontal axis.

3) Unequal class intervals should generally be avoided in constructing a histogram. Histograms are most commonly used for class intervals of equal size, because the area of each rectangle is proportional to the class frequency. If class intervals are unequal in size, the heights or widths must be adjusted. How this adjustment is done is not discussed in this text.

4) Generally, the horizontal axis represents the scores or class boundaries, with the midpoint of the interval in the center. The vertical axis generally represents the frequency.

Example: Thirty-six morbidly obese people were put on a controlled liquid diet for a month. Their weights were recorded at the beginning of the month and at the end of the month, and the difference between the initial weight and the final weight was recorded to the nearest pound. The number of pounds lost is as follows: 20, 12, 16, 24, 8, 22, 13, 22, 23, 22, 12, 15, 18, 14, 18, 10, 15, 27, 13, 26, 21, 14, 27, 11, 25, 22, 13, 17, 13, 11, 15, 17, 24, 17, 28, 20.

First a frequency distribution is constructed and then the histogram is graphed. Using a class interval size of two the frequency distribution would read:

Class Boundaries	Midpoint	Frequency
27.5 to 29.4	28.5	1
25.5 to 27.4	26.5	3
23.5 to 25.4	24.5	3
21.5 to 23.4	22.5	5
19.5 to 21.4	20.5	3
17.5 to 19.4	18.5	2
15.5 to 17.4	16.5	4
13.5 to 15.4	14.5	5
11.5 to 13.4	12.5	6
9.5 to 11.4	10.5	3
7.5 to 9.4	8.5	1

The histogram based on the above data would appear as follows:

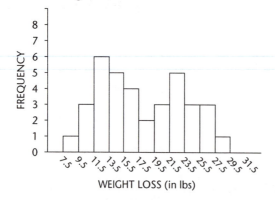

One-month weight loss on liquid diet (by a group of morbidly obese patients)

SELF-TEST 47: From the following frequency distribution, construct a histogram:

Systolic Blood Pressure	Midpoint	Frequency
89.5 to 109.4	99.5	16
109.5 to 129.4	119.5	37
129.5 to 149.4	139.5	29
149.5 to 169.4	159.5	12
169.5 to 189.4	179.5	4
189.5 to 209.4	199.5	2

*c. **Variations in Histogram Construction***

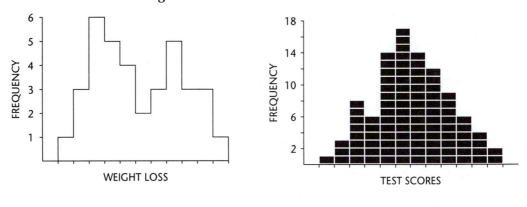

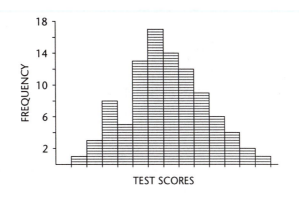

2. Frequency Polygon

A frequency polygon is similar to a histogram, in that it uses the same axes (horizontal and vertical) as the histogram and also is a graphic means of displaying continuous data. The plotting or graphic presentation differs, however, because a dot is placed at the frequency level on the vertical scale at the midpoint of the class interval. Instead of drawing rectangles, these points are connected by a straight line that is drawn from one point to the next point. To bring the figure to the baseline, dots are placed at the zero frequency level at the two ends of the distribution, extending the line to the horizontal at the midpoint of the lowest and highest interval.

a. Advantage of Frequency Polygon

The major advantage becomes apparent when similar data are compared. Frequency polygons can be superimposed on each other, which allows comparisons between the two data fields to be more readily made.

b. When to Use

Frequency polygons should only be used to graph quantitative (numerical) data and not qualitative data.

c. Construction of a Frequency Polygon

The frequency polygon is based on exactly the same information as is used to construct a histogram, but it displays quantitative data in a different graphic form. The frequency polygon may be considered a "connect-the-dots" diagram, because it joins adjacent frequencies by connecting straight lines.

To close the polygon at each end, a line is drawn to the baseline at the two ends of the distribution at the zero frequency level. At the upper end, the line extends from the frequency level of the upper interval to the horizontal (zero frequency level) where the next outlying interval occurs. This line is also extended to the baseline at the outlying lower level.

Example: Using the data from the frequency distribution referred to under the histogram example, the frequency polygon would be plotted as follows:

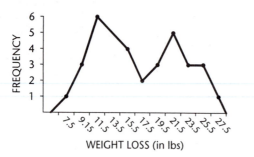

One-month weight loss on liquid diet (by a group of morbidly obese patients)

3. *Histogram and Frequency Polygon—Additional Information*

    a. Comparisons

        1) Similarities

            a) Same axes—horizontal and vertical—apply.

            b) Midpoints of class intervals are plotted.

            c) Graph the same type of data.

        2) Differences

            a) Points are plotted and connected rather than rectangles drawn to represent frequencies.

            b) A line is drawn to the baseline at the two ends to close a polygon.

    b. Supplementary Suggestions for Construction

        1) Limits

        Remember that the sides of the rectangles in a histogram are constructed along the class boundaries (real limits), whereas in a frequency polygon the frequency is indicated above the midpoint of the interval.

        2) Title

        Any graph or figure should always carry a complete, clear, and concise title. The title should completely identify the data represented. References to a graph should be made in the corresponding textual material, but the graph should *not* be dependent on any accompanying textual description.

        3) Labeling the Axes

        Vertical and horizontal axes should be clearly labeled and the scale units indicated.

    c. Superimposing Figures

    Data comparisons can be displayed by superimposing two frequency polygons on the same chart or graph. If two or more figures are drawn on the same chart, each should be distinguished differently. This could be done through the use of different colors for each figure or a variation in the typeset line drawn (solid, broken, dotted, etc.).

    A legend should be prominently placed (in the upper corner or another convenient space) to indicate the meaning of each of these variations to the reader.

    Example of a Superimposed Frequency Polygon: A comparison is to be made of the cholesterol levels of a group of 150 males and 150 females between the ages of 20 and 100. Included below is a frequency distribution of the cholesterol values, in which the scores ranged from a high of 415 to a low of 135. The distribution follows on the next page.

Cholesterol Values	Midpoint	Male Frequency	Female Frequency
399.5 to 419.4	409.5	1	0
379.5 to 399.4	389.5	0	1
359.5 to 379.4	369.5	2	0
339.5 to 359.4	349.5	3	2
319.5 to 339.4	329.5	2	2
299.5 to 319.4	309.5	4	2
279.5 to 299.4	289.5	3	2
259.5 to 279.4	269.5	5	5
239.5 to 259.4	249.5	8	5
219.5 to 239.4	229.5	22	18
199.5 to 219.4	209.5	35	45
179.5 to 199.4	189.5	21	27
159.5 to 179.4	169.5	24	30
139.5 to 159.4	149.5	18	10
119.5 to 139.4	129.5	2	1

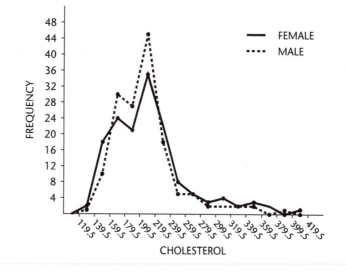

Male and female cholesterol levels (ages 20–100)

SELF-TEST 48: Construct a frequency polygon for the data in the Self-Test for the histogram on page 169.

4. *Bar Graph/Bar Chart*

The bar graph or bar chart is similar to the histogram. The major difference is in the type of data displayed. A bar graph is a convenient graphic device that is particularly useful for displaying qualitative data—such as ethnicity, sex, and treatment categories. A histogram, on the other hand, displays quantitative data that is continuous or discrete. (Discrete data is expressed as a whole number; continuous data is information that can be measured to the nearest whole number or a fraction—see page 4). The bar graph, in contrast, may compare data that cannot be measured in numbers—such as occupation or race. There often are no score limits along the horizontal axis. This type of graph is a convenient and useful means of displaying all kinds of numerical data—such as treatment modalities or the number of cases reported each month during a designated year.

a. *Construction of a Bar Graph*

Construction of the axes is similar to that used for the axes of the histogram. The horizontal axis consists of the various categories—such as modalities of treatment. The vertical axis again depicts the frequency or relative frequency. In this graph, however, the order of the categories along the horizontal axis may vary. It may be arranged:

1) alphabetically;
2) by frequency within a category; or
3) by using some other rational basis.

The height of each bar (rectangle) is based on the frequency for that category. Space is left between bars to alert the reader to the fact that no continuity is indicated and to reduce the possibility of implying that there is continuity.

The bars should be of equal width and stand apart from one another, as mentioned. Also, a broken line (or other means of interruption) should be used when the vertical axis does *not* begin at zero, as previously mentioned in the section on "Vertical Scale."

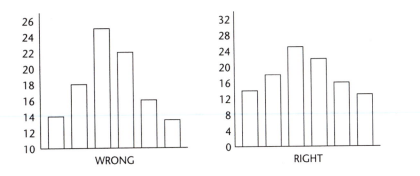

Example: A health department's records indicate the following number of reported and confirmed cases of sexually transmitted diseases during 1993:

Chlamydia	120	HSV-2	15
Trichomonas	90	Syphilis	3
Gonorrhea	45	AIDS	1
HPV	30		

A bar graph of these data would take the following form:

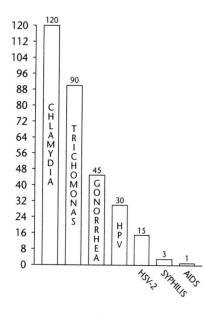

Sexually transmitted diseases reported in 1993 by the local Health Department

SELF-TEST 49: A hospital's records over the past decade revealed that the following number of patients have been treated for ectopic pregnancies:

1980	20	1985	31
1981	26	1986	28
1982	24	1987	27
1983	28	1988	32
1984	30	1989	31

Construct a bar graph using these data.

5. Line Graph

A line graph is to a bar graph what a frequency polygon is to a histogram. In other words, if the rectangle was replaced by a dot at the height of each frequency, and a line was drawn connecting these dots consecutively, the result would be a line graph.

Example: A hospital's records over the past decade showed the following yearly Cesarean section rates:

1980	44%	1985	35%
1981	42%	1986	33%
1982	38%	1987	35%
1983	38%	1988	30%
1984	35%	1989	27%

A line graph of these data would show the decrease as follows:

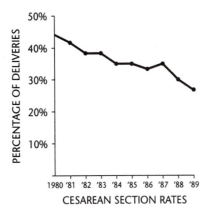

SELF-TEST 50: A hospital's records indicated the number of patients who delivered during the past ten years who were under the age of 16 at the time of delivery. Construct a line graph displaying these data:

1980	68	1985	166
1981	84	1986	182
1982	101	1987	203
1983	122	1988	210
1984	147	1989	241

6. Pie Graph/Pie Chart

Another common means of displaying data is a pie chart. A circle is divided into wedges in the same way that a pie is cut into slices for serving. Each wedge of the pie corresponds to the percentage of frequency of the distribution. Pie charts are useful in conveying data that consists of a small number of categories.

As with other graphs, be sure to clearly title the subject matter, to include dates if needed, and to indicate the percentages within each wedge and what the wedge represents.

Example: A tumor registrar has discovered the following percentages for female cancers:

Cervical   50.0%

Uterine   30.4%

Ovarian   16.5%

Vulvar   2.2%

Vaginal   0.9%

A pie chart of these data is as follows:

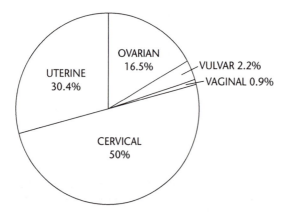

Female cancer

SELF-TEST 51: A hospital reports that, of the patients admitted over the age of 14 during the past year, the following percentages were reported regarding the patient's marital status at the time of admission to the hospital:

Single (never married)   18.8%

Married   55.2%

Widowed   10.5%

Divorced   15.5%

Develop a pie chart using these data.

7. Pictograph/Pictogram

Pictographs make use of pictures in their display of data. A common representative picture is a stick figure that represents a certain number of people. This is often used to present statistical data in a manner that is appealing to the general public. Pictograms often show great originality and ingenuity on the part of the presentor and, because they are eye-catching, can often draw the reader's attention to the data being displayed.

Example: Hospital records indicate that a total of 125 patients were admitted and given inpatient treatment for an infectious disease during the past year. The infections included the following:

Bacterial Infection	Frequency
Intestinal	49
TB (respiratory)	9
TB (non-respiratory)	4
Strep throat	7
Septicemia	14
Other bacteria	7

Viral Infection	Frequency
Exanthematous	7
Hepatitis	15
Other viral	24

The data are depicted below in pictograph form.

		Frequency
Bacterial:	Intestinal	49
	TB (respiratory)	9
	TB (non-respiratory)	4
	Strep throat	7
	Septicemia	14
	Other bacteria	7
Viral:	Viral (exanthematous)	7
	Viral hepatitis	15
	Other viral	24

Infections treated on an inpatient basis, 1993 (each figure represents 5 people)

8. Comparison Graph

Occasionally, two or more frequency distributions are plotted on the same graph using the same axes. This method is most commonly employed when comparisons are to be shown, especially between two related items. For example, you might choose to compare one hospital with another hospital, or one country with another country, and therefore plot both sets of data on the same graph. Comparisons are more easily seen when displayed in this fashion, instead of on two separate graphs, unless one can be laid directly over the other.

a. *Bar Graphs*

There are several ways by which two or more bar graphs can be compared, including the following:

1) Side-by-side comparisons.

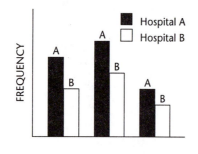

2) Component part graph (one on top of another).

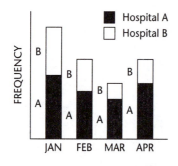

3) Percentage component part graph (on top of each other).

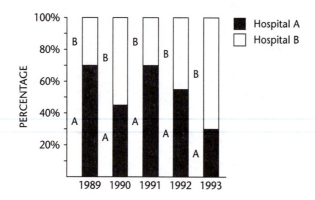

Example: A hospital wishes to compare (by month) the percentage of occupancy in 1993 with that in 1992. These were recorded as:

Month	1992	1993	Month	1992	1993
Jan.	85	78	July	75	72
Feb.	87	82	Aug.	78	70
Mar.	82	85	Sept.	80	75
Apr.	79	86	Oct.	82	72
May	75	80	Nov.	85	80
June	70	77	Dec.	73	80

The bar graph comparison would appear as follows:

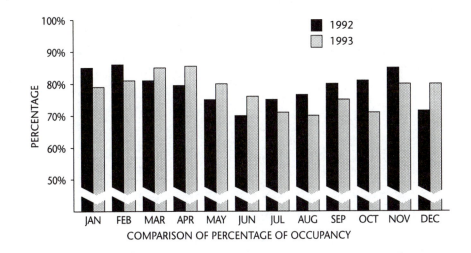

SELF-TEST 52: The local health department reports the following number of confirmed cases of measles and mumps over the past decade:

Year	Measles Frequency	Mumps Frequency
1980	13	9
1981	3	5
1982	1	5
1983	1	3
1984	3	3
1985	3	3
1986	6	8
1987	3	13
1988	3	5
1989	11	4

Construct a comparison bar graph for these data.

b. *Line Graphs*

The same rules that applied to superimposed frequency polygons hold true for line graphs. Each line should be distinguished differently, as previously mentioned. This could be accomplished by using different colors or a variation in the type of line drawn. Again, a legend should be included to indicate what each line represents.

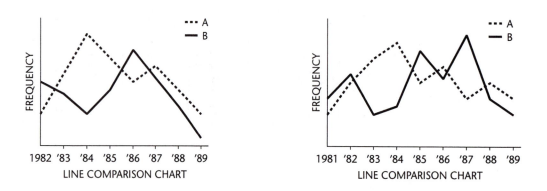

Example: A line graph comparison is to be made of the deaths recorded during 1991, comparing the number of male and female deaths.

Month	Male	Female	Month	Male	Female
Jan.	19	17	July	22	15
Feb.	13	15	Aug.	25	22
Mar.	20	12	Sept.	20	24
Apr.	15	18	Oct.	18	22
May	18	15	Nov.	19	20
June	21	12	Dec.	24	18

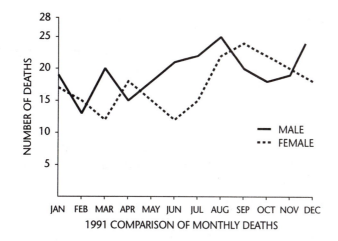

1991 COMPARISON OF MONTHLY DEATHS

SELF-TEST 53: Construct a comparison line graph of the measles and mumps data from the previous section (on bar graphs).

C. SUMMARY

The following general rules apply to graphs:
1. Graphs convey information more quickly than tables do.
2. Graphs are generally more impressive than tables.
3. Graphs should relate sufficient information so that the reader does not need to refer to textual material, although additional information regarding the data may be made available in the accompanying text.
4. Graphs should be simple, clear, and uncomplicated so that the message is readily apparent to the viewer.
5. Appropriate and descriptive titles should accompany all graphs. The title should inform the reader about what is being graphed and/or compared, the time period or the dates during which the data was collected, and the source of the data (the group on which the data was collected).

D. CHAPTER 11 TEST

1. For each of the variables listed below, circle the more appropriate graphical method to use to display it.
   a. Number of x-rays performed per person.   Histogram   Bar Graph
   b. Triglyceride level of 100 patients.   Freq. Polygon   Line Graph

   c. Percentage classification of patients   Histogram   Pie Chart
       by occupation.
   d. Birth rate comparison by years.   Freq. Polygon   Line Graph

2. When plotting a histogram, what is most commonly plotted along the
   a. horizontal axis?

   b. vertical axis?

3. One hundred forty-one cases of CHD (coronary heart disease) have been recently diagnosed. Of these, 83 were males and 58 were females. The ages at the time of initial diagnosis were distributed as follows:

Score Limits	Midpoint	Male Freq.	Female Freq.
80–84	82	5	6
75–79	77	5	4
70–74	72	7	11
65–69	67	17	11
60–64	62	20	12
55–59	57	11	5
50–54	52	6	4
45–49	47	4	2
40–44	42	3	2
35–39	37	2	0
30–34	32	1	1
25–29	27	2	0

Calculate:

a. Mean age at time of diagnosis of CHD from the grouped frequency distribution for
   1) all patients.

   2) all male patients.

   3) all female patients.

b. Construct a comparison histogram of the age differences for the two sexes.

4. Comparative admission statistics for 1985 to 1989 were as follows:

Month	1985	1986	1987	1988	1989	Month	1985	1986	1987	1988	1989
Jan.	661	531	472	463	460	July	563	542	547	481	455
Feb.	572	470	474	472	480	Aug.	546	551	530	421	406
Mar.	583	526	482	480	466	Sept.	484	493	505	458	463
Apr.	560	493	424	512	501	Oct.	533	538	508	437	424
May	546	562	446	538	498	Nov.	558	472	442	438	427
June	487	558	462	484	460	Dec.	547	503	478	439	410

Construct a comparative line graph of the above data.

5. A hospital recorded the twelve most commonly reported cancers during the past year and the percentage of males and females diagnosed with each type as follows:

Cancer Site	Male Percentage	Female Percentage
Lung	66%	34%
Colorectal	48%	52%
Breast	1%	99%
Prostate	100%	–
Urinary tract	70%	30%
Uterine	–	100%
Oral	68%	32%
Leukemia	56%	44%
Pancreatic	50%	50%
Skin	53%	47%
Stomach	61%	39%
Ovarian	–	100%

Construct a percentage component part graph of these data.

6. In reviewing the newly diagnosed cancer cases over the past year, the cancer registrar reported the following:

Cancer Site	Percentage of Total Cases
Lung	16
Colorectal	15
Breast	14
Prostate	10
Urinary tract	7
Uterine	5
Oral	3
Leukemia	2.7
Skin	2.7
Stomach	2.5
Ovarian	2
Other	20.1

Construct a pie graph of these percentages.

7. A record is kept of the most common inpatient ENT procedures and the number of cases of each performed over the past six months. These are recorded as follows:

Procedure	*Number of Cases*
Tonsillectomy with Adenoidectomy	147
Tonsillectomy without Adenoidectomy	42
Septoplasty	16
Sialadenectomy (all types)	16
Mastoidectomy (all types)	15
Myringotomy with insertion of tube	14
Laryngoscopy/Tracheoscopy	12
Myringoplasty	7
Ethmoidectomy	7
Laryngectomy (radical)	7
Epistaxis control	6
Thyroidectomy (all types)	5
Stapedectomy	5
Pharyngoplasty	5
Rhinoplasty (all types)	4
Dacryocystorhinostomy	3

Construct a pictograph of these data.

Exam—Chapters 9 through 11

Note: Compute all required computations correct to *two* decimal places.

1. Thirty-five deaths (17 males and 18 females) have been reported during the past year. The ages of the patients at the time of death are as follows:

Males:	68	82	33	44	73	59	57	51	2	62	47
	46	48	70	80	37	59					

Females:	45	82	52	68	76	59	59	55	36	65	66
	52	84	63	46	24	80	NB				

Calculate:

a. Mean age at the time of death of

  1) all patients.

  2) all male patients.

  3) all female patients.

  4) all female patients if the newborn is excluded.

  5) all patients if the newborn is excluded.

b. Median age of all 35 patients at the time of death.

c. Mode of the distribution.

Construct:

d. A frequency distribution of all the ages using the following score limits, with a separate column for males and females:

Score Limits	Midpoint	Frequency	Cumulative Frequency
100+			
90–99			
80–89			
70–79			
60–69			
50–59			
40–49			
30–39			
20–29			
10–19			
0–9			

Indicate:

e. The size of a class interval.

Calculate:

f. Mean from the grouped frequency distribution.

Construct:

g. A comparison chart, comparing the ages of death of males and females, for the grouped frequency distribution.

2. Construct a comparison bar graph of the following data:

	Deaths	
Year	Under 48 hours	Over 48 hours
1989	72	253
1990	68	278
1991	64	268
1992	58	254
1993	52	246

3. Construct a percentage component part graph of autopsy rates, comparing the percentage of deaths that were unautopsied versus those that were autopsied or were coroner's cases.

Year	Deaths	Unautopsied	%	Autopsies	%	Coroner	%
1989	312	247	79	58	19	7	2
1990	344	281	82	52	15	11	3
1991	338	273	81	55	16	10	3
1992	310	264	85	41	13	5	2
1993	323	272	84	47	15	4	1

4. Construct a frequency distribution of the lengths of stay (in days) of patients at least one year old who underwent neurosurgery, using a class interval size of 2.

LOS:	13	4	7	2	2	5	4	7	6	11
	33	5	5	3	7	4	1	3	6	1
	20	3	3	4	5	3	4	7	6	6
	21	2	2	1	3	4	3	2	1	
	14	1	9	2	2	2	4	3	6	
	16	4	6	7	2	2	7	1	3	
	14	1	3	1	5	3	4	3	3	
	13	5	2	4	4	2	2	6	5	

Calculate:

a. Mean of the original, ungrouped lengths of stay.

b. Mean of the grouped lengths of stay.

c. Median of the ungrouped data.

d. Mode of the distribution.

Approximate:

e. Percentile rank of

    1) a length of stay of 16 days.

    2) a length of stay of 9 days.

Calculate:

f. Range of the distribution.

Construct:

g. A histogram of the data in this frequency distribution.

5. The ages of pediatric surgery patients (a total of 80 patients) were recorded as follows:

Ages:	*Years*				*Months*	*Days*	
	14	2	5	7	11	1	4
	12	8	1	4	7	25	5
	5	1	2	2	11	4	7
	3	5	1	6	10	21	4
	12	1	1	7	7	5	4
	9	4	8	2	9	27	3
	11	1	7	5	5	18	5
	11	3	2	3	9	6	4
	10	3	9	3	2	1	1
	14	5	1	3	1	1	1
	10	2	4	8	7	1	1
	3	1				1	

Calculate:

a. Mean of the ungrouped ages, assuming there are 30 days in an average month.

b. Median of the ungrouped age distribution.

c. Mode of the entire ungrouped distribution.

d. Mean age of the ungrouped patients at least one year old.

e. Mean age of the ungrouped patients less than one month old.

f. Median age of the ungrouped patients less than one month old.

g. Mode of the ungrouped patients less than one month old.

h. Mode of the ungrouped patients at least one year old.

6. Semiannual surgical records reveal the following number of surgical procedures performed on inpatients, and their respective percentages.

Procedure by Medical Specialty	Number of Procedures	Percentage
Cardiovasular	62	15
Oncology	7	2
Thoracic/Pulmonary	11	2.5
ENT	11	2.5
General surgery	111	27
Neurosurgery	4	1
Orthopedic surgery	78	19
Urology	27	6.5
OB	28	7
Gynecologic surgery	40	10
Newborn surgery	31	7.5

Construct a pie graph to represent these data.

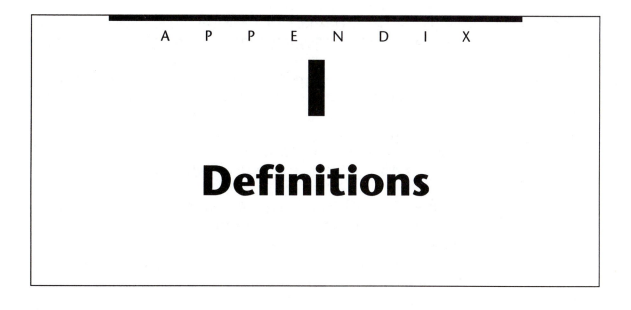

APPENDIX

I

Definitions

There are a variety of terms used in health care facilities that are related to or relevant to statistics. The majority of these terms have been used throughout this manual and are included here for easy reference.

A. PATIENT TERMS

Hospital Patient: An individual who receives, in person, hospital-based or hospital-coordinated medical services for which the hospital is responsible.

Hospital Inpatient: A hospital patient who is provided with room, board, and continuous general nursing service in an area of the hospital where patients generally stay at least overnight.

Hospital Newborn Inpatient: A hospital patient who was born in the hospital at the beginning of his current inpatient hospitalization.

Hospital Boarder: An individual who receives lodging in the hospital but who is not a hospital inpatient.

Pediatric Patient: A patient who is usually under the age of 14. No general agreement exists on the age at which a patient is no longer a child (pediatric patient) and is considered an adult. The dividing line is most often drawn at the 14th birthday, so patients 13 years old or younger are considered pediatric patients. The American Hospital Association (AHA) defines "pediatric service" as the diagnosis and treatment of patients usually under the age of 14.

Hospital Outpatient: A hospital patient who receives service in one or more of the facilities of the hospital at a time when he is currently neither an inpatient nor a home care patient.

B. INPATIENT TERMS

Inpatient Hospitalization: A single hospital stay as an inpatient without interruption, except for possible intervening leaves of absence.

Inpatient Admission: The formal acceptance by a hospital of a patient who is to be provided with room, board, and continuous nursing service in an area of the hospital where patients generally stay overnight.

Inpatient Discharge: The termination of a period of inpatient hospitalization through the formal release of the inpatient by the hospital (end of a hospitalization). A discharge includes any of the following:

1. Released by order of the physician.
2. Left against medical advice (abbreviated AMA).
3. Transferred to another facility—hospital, nursing home, etc.
4. Death of the patient.

(The term discharge includes deaths; however, if the term "live discharges" is used, deaths must be added to these discharges to determine the total discharges.)

Day on Leave of Absence: A day occurring after the admission and prior to the discharge of a hospital inpatient, during which the patient is not present at the census-taking hour because he is on leave of absence from the hospital.

Transfers:
Intrahospital—a change in the medical care unit of an inpatient during hospitalization.
Interhospital (Discharge Transfer)—the relocation of an inpatient to another health care institution at the time of discharge.

C. CENSUS-RELATED TERMS

Census: Count; an official count of people.

Inpatient Census: The number of patients present at any one time.

Daily Inpatient Census (DIPC): The number of patients present at the census-taking time each day *plus* any inpatients who were admitted and discharged (A&D) after the census-taking time the previous day.

Inpatient Service Day (IPSD): A unit of measure denoting the services received by one inpatient during one 24-hour period.

Total Inpatient Service Days: The sum of all the inpatient service days for each of the days during the period under consideration.

Average Daily Inpatient Census (Average Daily Census): Average number of inpatients present each day for a given period of time.

D. BED/BASSINET COUNT TERMS

Inpatient Bed Count/Bed Complement: The number of available hospital inpatient beds, both occupied and vacant, on any given day.

Newborn Bassinet Count: The number of available hospital newborn bassinets, both occupied and vacant, on a given day.

Inpatient Bed Count Day: A unit of measure denoting the presence of one inpatient bed, set up and staffed for use, and either occupied or vacant, during one 24-hour period.

Inpatient Bassinet Count Day: A unit of measure denoting the presence of one inpatient bassinet, set up and staffed for use, and either occupied or vacant, during one 24-hour period.

Inpatient Bed Count Days (Total): The sum of inpatient bed count days for each of the days during the period under consideration.

E. OCCUPANCY TERMS

Inpatient Bed Occupancy Ratio: The proportion of inpatient beds occupied, defined as the ratio of service days to inpatient bed count days during the period under consideration.

F. DEATH-RELATED TERMS

Anesthesia Death: Death caused by an anesthetic agent.

Postoperative Death: Surgical death within ten days after an operation.

Maternal Death: Death of any woman from any cause, while pregnant or within 42 days of termination of pregnancy, irrespective of the duration and the site of the pregnancy.

Direct Maternal Death: Death directly related to pregnancy.

Indirect Material Death: Maternal death not directly due to obstetric causes but aggravated by the pregnant condition.

Hospital Fetal Death: Death prior to the complete expulsion or extraction from its mother, in a hospital facility, of a product of human conception, fetus and placenta, irrespective of the duration of pregnancy. The death is indicated by the fact that, after such expulsion or extraction, the fetus does not breathe or show any other evidence of life, such as beating of the heart, pulsation of the umbilical cord, or definite movement of voluntary muscles.

   Early Fetal Death: Fetal deaths under 20 weeks of gestation (and weighing 500 grams or less); also referred to as "abortion."

   Intermediate Fetal Death: Fetal deaths in which the fetus has completed 20 of weeks gestation but less than 28 weeks of gestation (and weighing 501 to 1000 grams).

   Late Fetal Death: Fetal deaths in which the fetus has completed 28 weeks of gestation (and is 1001 grams or more in weight); also referred to as "stillbirth."

Stillborn Infant: A fetus, irrespective of its gestational age, that after complete expulsion or extraction . . . shows no evidence of life (as delineated above).

Perinatal Death: An all-inclusive term referring to both stillborn infants and neonatal deaths.

Neonatal Death: Death of a liveborn infant within the first 27 days, 23 hours, and 59 minutes from the moment of birth. (This is also the period during which an infant is considered a newborn.)

Infant Death: Death of a liveborn infant at any time from the moment of birth to the end of the first year of life (364 days, 23 hours, and 59 minutes from the moment of birth).

G. AUTOPSY TERMS

Autopsy: Inspection and partial dissection of a dead body to learn the cause of death, and the nature and extent of disease; postmortem examination.

Hospital Inpatient Autopsy: Postmortem examination performed in a hospital facility, by a hospital pathologist or by a physician on the medical staff to whom the responsibility has been delegated, on the body of a patient who died during inpatient hospitalization.

Hospital Autopsy: Postmortem examination performed by a hospital pathologist or by a physician on the medical staff to whom the responsibility has been delegated, wherever performed, and regardless of the hospitalization status of the patient at the time of his death.

Available for Hospital Autopsy: The body of a current or former hospital patient that has been transported to the appropriate facility for autopsy. This also includes that the

1. necessary authorization is given by the patient's relatives;
2. hospital pathologist has agreed to perform the autopsy;
3. autopsy report will be filed in the patient's hospital medical record and in the hospital laboratory;
4. tissue specimens will be maintained in the hospital laboratory.

H. LENGTH OF STAY/DISCHARGE DAY TERMS

Length of Stay (for one patient): The number of calendar days from admission to discharge.

Total Length of Stay (for all patients): The sum of the days of stay of any group of inpatients discharged during a specified period of time.

I. OB/MATERNAL TERMS (excluding those related to death)

Obstetrics: All patients having diseases and conditions of pregnancy, labor, and the puerperium, whether normal or pathological.

Puerperium: The period of 42 days following delivery; this period is included as part of the pregnancy period.

Delivery: Expelling of a product of conception or having it removed from the body. Multiple births are considered a single delivery. A delivery may include either a live infant or a dead fetus.

Delivered in the Hospital: Includes mothers for whom the pregnancy has terminated in the hospital, regardless of whether the infant is liveborn or is a fetal death.

Admitted After Delivery: Includes mothers for whom the pregnancy terminated before reaching the hospital, regardless of whether the infant is liveborn or is a fetal death. These patients are often included under the category "not delivered."

Aborted: Includes mothers for whom the pregnancy has terminated in less than the time specified by the health agency for a viable infant. It includes the expulsion or extraction of all or any part of the placenta or membranes without an identifiable fetus or with a liveborn infant or a stillborn weighing less than 500 grams or occurring before the 20th completed week of gestation.

Pregnancy Termination: Expulsion or extraction of a dead fetus or other products of conception from the mother, or the birth of a liveborn infant or a stillborn infant.

Induced Termination of Pregnancy: The purposeful interruption of an intrauterine pregnancy, with the intention being other than to produce a liveborn infant, and which does not result in a live birth.

Not Delivered: Includes pregnant women admitted for a condition of pregnancy but not delivered of a liveborn or stillborn infant in the hospital. (The women may have been admitted because of threatened abortion or false labor.)

J. NEWBORN TERMS (excluding terms related to newborn deaths)

Hospital Live Birth: The complete expulsion or extraction from the mother, in a hospital facility, of a product of human conception, irrespective of the duration of pregnancy, which, after such expulsion or extraction, breathes or shows any other evidence of life, such as beating of the heart, pulsation of the umbilical cord, or definite movement of voluntary muscles, whether or not the umbilical cord has been cut or the placenta is attached. Heartbeats are to be distinguished from transient cardiac contractions; respirations are to be distinguished from fleeting respiratory efforts or gasps.

Premature Birth: Newborn with a birthweight of less than 2500 grams (5 lb 3 oz).

Neonatal Periods:

Period I: From hour of birth through 23 hours and 59 minutes.
Period II: From beginning of 24th hour through 6 days, 23 hours, and 59 minutes.
Period III: From beginning of 7th day through 27 days, 23 hours, 59 minutes.

K. MISCELLANEOUS TERMS

Medical Services: The activities related to the medical care performed by physicians, nurses, and other professional and technical personnel under the direction of a physician.

Medical Staff Unit: One of the departments, divisions, or specialties into which the organized medical staff of a hospital is divided in order to fulfill medical staff responsibilities.

Medical Care Unit: An assemblage of inpatient beds (or newborn bassinets) and related facilities and assigned personnel in which medical services are provided to a defined and limited class of patients according to their particular medical care needs.

Special Care Unit: A medical care unit in which there is appropriate equipment and a concentration of physicians, nurses, and others who have special skills and experience to provide optimal medical care for critically ill patients, or continuous care of patients in special diagnostic categories.

Surgical Procedure: Any single, separate, systematic manipulation upon or within the body that can be complete in itself, normally performed by a physician, dentist, or other licensed practitioner, either with or without instruments, to restore disunited or deficient parts, to remove diseased or injured tissues, to extract foreign matter, to assist in obstetrical delivery, or to aid in diagnosis.

Surgical Operation: One or more surgical procedures performed at one time for one patient using a common approach or for a common purpose.

Medical Consultation: The response by one member of the medical staff to a request for consultation by another member of the medical staff, characterized by review of the patient's history, examination of the patient, and completion of a consultation report that gives recommendations and/or opinions.

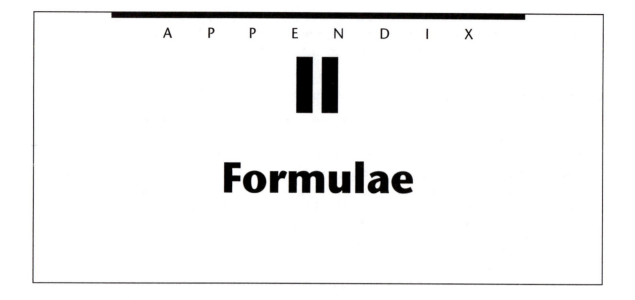

A P P E N D I X

II

Formulae

Listed below are the basic formulae used for hospital statistics. They have been included in the various chapters of the text and are repeated here for easy reference.

A. CENSUS FORMULAE

Inpatient Census: Patients remaining at the previous census-taking time *plus* addition of new admissions and subtraction of the day's discharges (including the deaths).

Inpatient Service Days: Census plus A&Ds (those admitted and discharged the same day).

Average DIPC:

$$\frac{\text{Total IPSD for a period}}{\text{Total number of days in the period}}$$

A&C Average DIPC:

$$\frac{\text{Total IPSD (excluding NB) for a period}}{\text{Total number of days in the period}}$$

NB Average DIPC:

$$\frac{\text{Total NB IPSD for a period}}{\text{Total number of days in the period}}$$

Clinical Unit Average DIPC:

$$\frac{\text{Total IPSD for the clinical unit for a period}}{\text{Total number of days in the period}}$$

B. RATE FORMULA

$$\frac{\text{Number of times something happens}}{\text{Number of times it could happen}}$$

C. OCCUPANCY FORMULAE

Daily IP Bed Occupancy Percentage:

$$\frac{\text{Daily IPSD}}{\text{IP bed count for that day}} \times 100$$

Daily NB Bassinet Occupancy Percentage:

$$\frac{\text{Daily NB IPSD}}{\text{NB bassinet count for that day}} \times 100$$

IP Bed Occupancy Percentage for a Period:

$$\frac{\text{Total IPSD for a period}}{\text{Total IP bed count days} \times \text{number of days in period}} \times 100$$

NB Bassinet Occupancy Percentage for a Period:

$$\frac{\text{Total NB IPSD for a period}}{\text{Total NB bassinet count} \times \text{number of days in period}} \times 100$$

Clinical Unit Occupancy Percentage for a Period:

$$\frac{\text{Total IPSD in a clinical unit for a period}}{\text{IP bed count total for that unit} \times \text{number of days in period}} \times 100$$

Occupancy Percentage for a Period with a Change in Bed Count:

$$\frac{\text{Total IPSD for the period}}{(\text{Bed count} \times \text{days}) + (\text{Bed count} \times \text{days})} \times 100$$

(Days refers to number of days in the period.)

D. DEATH RATES

1. General

Gross Death Rate:

$$\frac{\text{Total number of deaths (including NB) for a period}}{\text{Total number of discharges for the period (including deaths of NB + A\&C)}} \times 100$$

Net Death Rate:

$$\frac{\text{Total IP deaths (+ NB)} - \text{deaths} <48 \text{ hrs for a period}}{\text{Total discharges} - \text{deaths} <48 \text{ hrs for the period}} \times 100$$

NB Death Rate:

$$\frac{\text{Total NB deaths for a period}}{\text{Total NB discharges for the period}} \times 100$$

2. **Surgical Death Rates**

Postoperative Death Rate:

$$\frac{\text{Total surgical deaths <10 days postop for period}}{\text{Total patients operated upon for the period}} \times 100$$

Anesthesia Death Rate:

$$\frac{\text{Total deaths caused by anesthetic agents for period}}{\text{Total number of anesthesias administered for the period}} \times 100$$

3. **Maternal/Fetal Death Rates**

Maternal Death Rate:

$$\frac{\text{Total maternal deaths for a period}}{\text{Total maternal discharges for a period (including deaths)}} \times 100$$

Fetal Death Rate:

$$\frac{\text{Total number of intermediate and late fetal deaths for period}}{\substack{\text{Total number of births for the period} \\ \text{(including live births, intermediate and late fetal deaths)}}} \times 100$$

E. AUTOPSY RATES

Gross Autopsy Rate:

$$\frac{\text{Total autopsies on IP deaths for a period}}{\text{Total IP deaths}} \times 100$$

Net Autopsy Rate:

$$\frac{\text{Total autopsies on IP deaths for a period}}{\text{Total IP deaths – unautopsied coroner's cases}} \times 100$$

Hospital Autopsy Rate:

$$\frac{\text{Total number of hospital autopsies for period}}{\substack{\text{Number of deaths of hospital patients whose bodies are available for} \\ \text{hospital autopsy for that period}}} \times 100$$

NB Autopsy Rate:

$$\frac{\text{Autopsies on NB deaths for period}}{\text{Total NB deaths for period}} \times 100$$

Fetal Autopsy Rate:

$$\frac{\text{Autopsies on intermediate and late fetal deaths for period}}{\text{Total intermediate and late fetal deaths for period}} \times 100$$

F. OTHER RATES

Cesarean Section Rate:

$$\frac{\text{Total C-sections performed in a period}}{\text{Total number of deliveries for the period}} \times 100$$

Hospital Infection Rate:

$$\frac{\text{Total number of infections}}{\text{Total number of discharges (including deaths)}}$$

Consultation Rate:

$$\frac{\text{Total number of consultations performed}}{\text{Total number of discharges (including deaths)}}$$

Postoperative Infection Rate:

$$\frac{\text{Total number of postoperative infections}}{\text{Total number of surgical operations}}$$

Bed/Bassinet Turnover Rate—Direct formula:

$$\frac{\text{Total number of discharges (including deaths) for a period}}{\text{Average bed count during the period}}$$

Bed/Bassinet Turnover Rate—Indirect formula:

$$\frac{\text{Occupancy rate} \times \text{number of days in the period}}{\text{Average length of stay}}$$

G. LENGTH OF STAY

Average Length of Stay:

$$\frac{\text{Total discharge days (+ deaths but excluding NB)}}{\text{Total discharges (+ deaths but excluding NB)}}$$

Average NB Length of Stay:

$$\frac{\text{Total NB discharge days (+ deaths)}}{\text{Total NB discharges (+ deaths)}}$$

III

Answer Key

CHAPTER 1

Chapter 1 Test

1. a. Population
   b. Sample
   c. Population
2. a. Variable
   b. Constant
3. a. Quantitative
   b. Qualitative
   c. Qualitative
   d. Quantitative
   e. Quantitative
   f. Qualitative
   g. Quantitative
   h. Qualitative
4. a. Discrete
   b. Continuous
   c. Discrete
   d. Continuous
   e. Discrete
   f. Discrete
   g. Continuous
5. a. 91-88-84-81-80-80-77-77-77-73-73-73-72-
      67-66-66-65-63-62-61-59-59 59-58-58-56-56-
      55-55-51-49-49-48-48-47-47-44-42-39-38-37-
      37-33-28-27-27-21-18

b.

Score	Tally	Score	Tally
91	/	56	//
88	/	55	//
84	/	51	/
81	/	49	//
80	//	48	//
77	///	47	//
73	///	44	/
72	/	42	/
67	/	39	/
66	//	38	/
65	/	37	//
63	/	33	/
62	/	28	/
61	/	27	//
59	///	21	/
58	//	18	/

c.

94-97	-	66-69	///		
90-93	/	62-65	///	38-41	//
86-89	/	58-61	//////	34-37	//
82-85	/	54-57	////	30-33	/
78-81	///	50-53	/	26-29	///
74-77	///	46-49	//////	22-25	-
70-73	////	42-45	//	18-21	//

6. a. newborn
   b. summation sign
   c. admitted and discharged (the same day)
   d. adults and children
   e. dead on arrival
   f. inpatient
   g. length of stay
   h. intensive care unit

CHAPTER 2

Self-Tests

1. **Fractions:**
   Caucasian, 43/85; African American, 25/85 or 5/17; Hispanic, 12/85; Oriental, 5/85 or 1/17

2. **Numerator:**
   a. 3
   b. 10
   c. 6

3. **Denominator:**
   a. 17
   b. 10
   c. 8

4. **Quotient:**
   a. 2.22
   b. 0.78
   c. 0.72

5. **Decimals:**
   a. 0.05
   b. 0.007
   c. 0.01

6. **Percentage:**
   a. 6%
   b. 50%
   c. 0.8%
   d. 56%

7. **Rates:**
   5/120 or 4%

8. **Ratio:**
   Orthopedic, 20/100 or 20%
   Gynecological, 12/100 or 12%
   Ophthalmological, 18/100 or 18%
   Urological, 22/100 or 22%
   General surgery, 28/100 or 28%

9. **Averaging:**
   1. 8   4. 6
   2. 4   5. 2
   3. 19

10. **Rounding:**
    1. a. 65   e. 7051   i. 148
       b. 66   f. 1   j. 10
       c. 66   g. 38   k. 16
       d. 71   h. 596   l. 56
    2. a. 12.4   e. 457.0   i. 6.6
       b. 27.6   f. 699.0   j. 76.0
       c. 31.7   g. 84.0
       d. 0.0   h. 1.1
    3. a. 65.70   e. 126.00   i. 100.06
       b. 68.64   f. 65.67   j. 1.15
       c. 0.01   g. 18.00
       d. 953.80 h. 80.00

4. a. 3300   e. 4,000,000
   b. 5.8   f. 2180
   c. 0.005   g. 43.88
   d. 46.74   h. 46,000

11. **Fraction to Percentage:**
    a. 66.7%
    b. 50%
    c. 10%
    d. 41.0%
    e. 62.5%

12. **Ratio to Percentage:**
    a. 33%
    b. 64%
    c. 83%
    d. 65%
    e. 25%

13. **Decimal to Percentage:**
    1. a. 125%   e. 0.6%
       b. 63.5%   f. 82.35%
       c. 30%   g. 1.62%
       d. 3%   h. 55%
    2. a. 325%   d. 56%
       b. 46%   e. 2%
       c. 1%   f. 4%

14. **Percentage to Decimal:**
    a. 0.05   c. 0.005
    b. 0.114   d. 1.25

15. **Percentage to Fraction:**
    a. 3/4   e. 1/5
    b. 7/8   f. 84/100 = 21/25
    c. 1/3   g. 1/2
    d. 9/8   h. 98/100 = 49/50

16. **Computing with a Percentage:**
    1. 1/4   6. 0.12
    2. 5/8   7. 420
    3. 3/5   8. 67
    4. 0.005   9. 23
    5. 0.03   10. 46

Chapter 2 Test

1. a. 4.6 days
   b. 12.4 cases
   c. 10 autopsies
2. a. 40.64   d. 11.00
   b. 40.67   e. 18.56
   c. 40.70   f. 0.10
3. a. 40   d. 7770
   b. 71   e. 1
   c. 68   f. 56
4. a. 4500   d. 5,000,000   g. 87,000
   b. 4.7   e. 63.90
   c. 0.006   f. 80

5. a. 75%   d. 66%   g. 12%
   b. 40%   e. 108%   h. 66.7%
   c. 3%   f. 87.5%
6. a. 3/5   d. 1/3
   b. 4/5   e. 1/10
   c. 7/13   f. 1/20
7. a. 0.08   d. 0.73
   b. 0.13   e. 0.11
   c. 0.69   f. 1.00
8. a. 5076
   b. 87
   c. 5055

CHAPTER 3

Self-Tests

17. Census:
  1. a. 469
     b. 475
     c. 475
  2. 23
  3. a. 99
     b. 102
     c. 102
  4. a. 151
     b. 152
     c. 152
  5. a. 1250
     b. 47
     c. 379
     d. 42

18. Average Census:
  1. Jan–Apr 364.375
    May–Aug 481.447
    Sept–Dec 535.926
  2. a. 256.06
     b. 238.06
     c. 18
  3. a. A&C = 135; NB = 7
     b. A&C = 141.2
     c. NB = 13.7
  4. a. Ped = 11.5; Ortho = 14.4; Psych = 9.5
     b. Ped = 8; Ortho = 11; Psych = 7
     c. 1061

Chapter 3 Test

1. Daily inpatient census includes A&Ds.
2. Number of days in the period.
3. Same time each day.
4. a. No
  b. Yes
5. Unit B

6. a. Born and died the same day.
  b. Transferred to another hospital the same day.
  c. Discharged the day of birth.
7. a. A&C = 146; NB = 11
  b. Same as a.
  c. A&C = 148; NB = 11
  d. Same as c.
8. a. Urology, 17; ENT, 15; Ophth, 22
  b. 1526
  c. Urology, 16.7; ENT, 13.9; Ophth, 20.2
9. a. 55
  b. 660
  c. 60
  d. 1712
  e. 55.2
10. a. 469
   b. 475
   c. 475
11. 19
12. 99.8
13. 15
14. a. 127
   b. 129
   c. 129
15. a. 151
   b. 154
   c. 151
   d. 154

CHAPTER 4

Self-Tests

19. Percentage of Occupancy:
  1.   61.7%
  2.   70.6%
  3.   106.7%
  4.   96.2%
  5.   86.7%
  6. a. 7
     b. 58.3%

20. Occupancy for a Period:
  1. a. Dec. 1 thru Dec. 10
     b. 90.86%
  2. August thru October
  3. a. 96%
     b. February 4 and February 19
     c. 87.86%
     d. February 15 thru 21; 90.29%
  4. a. 92.38%
     b. 11
  5. a. Medical, 95%

Surgical, 96.86%
Pediatric, 93.78%
Orthopedic, 92.96%
Obstetric, 90.67%
Newborn, 97.04% = Best
  b. 94.58%
21. Change in Count:
  1. a. Jan. thru Mar.   95.42%
     Apr. thru June   96.07%
     July thru Sept.   96.65%
     Oct. thru Dec.   96.22%
    b. Jan. thru Mar.   93.67%
     Apr. thru June   90.99%
     July thru Sept.   90.54%
     Oct. thru Dec.   94.78%
    c. 96.12%
    d. 92.43%
    e. July thru Sept.
  2. 81.57%
  3. 95.32%
  4. 95.89%
  5. a. 98.39%
    b. 94.07%
    c. 93.72%
    d. 91.57%
    e. 95.22%
    f. 93.63%
    g. Oct. thru Dec.
    h. Apr. thru June
  6. a. 96.26%
    b. 85.92%

Chapter 4 Test
  1. a. 84.96%
    b. 96.92%
    c. May 1 thru May 10   75.23%
     May 11 thru May 20   86.62%
     May 21 thru May 31   92.31%
    d. 78.71%
  2. a. 99%
    b. 90%
    c. 76%
    d. A&C = 97
     NB = 9
     Surg = 19
  3. a. 14
    b. 15
    c. 93.75%
  4. a. Bed percentage:
     Jan. thru Mar.   86.15%
     Apr. thru June   89.26%

July thru Sept.   85.74%
Oct. thru Dec.   92.01%
Bassinet percentage:
  Jan. thru Mar.   85.06%
  Apr. thru June   91.36%
  July thru Sept.   87.77%
  Oct. thru Dec.   90.61%
Surgical unit percentage:
  Jan. thru Mar.   96.89%
  Apr. thru June   92.16%
  July thru Sept.   94.24%
  Oct. thru Dec.   90.47%
  b. Surgical = 93.16%
  5. a. 80.56%
    b. 86.45%
    c. 74.73%
  6. a. Medical   95.40%
     Surgical   92.29%
     Pediatrics   71.67%
     Orthopedics   92.22%
     Ophthalmology   93.60%
     Obstetrics   90.00%
     Newborn   90.00%
    b. 92.11%
    c. 91.96%
  7. a. Bed occupancy percentage:
     Jan. 1 thru Feb. 15 92.15%
     Feb. 16 thru Mar. 31 92.70%
     Apr. 1 thru Apr. 30 90.48%
     May 1 thru June 10 77.55%
    Bassinet occupancy percentage:
     Jan. 1 thru Feb. 15   83.88%
     Feb. 16 thru Mar. 31   89.20%
     Apr. 1 thru Apr. 30   90.67%
     May 1 thru June 10   82.90%
    b. Bed: 87.52%
     Bassinet: 85.37%
    c. Period B (Feb. 16 thru Mar. 31)
  8. a. 80.65%
    b. 94.98%
    c. 91.57%
    d. 96.02%
    e. 93.66%
    f. Last quarter
  9. a. 1250
    b. 379
    c. 38.90
    d. 41.67
    e. 83.33%
    f. 104%
    g. 79.11%

CHAPTER 5

Self-Tests

22. Gross/Net/Newborn Deaths

1. a. 5.5%
   b. 4.6%
   c. 8.3%
2. a. 7.9%
   b. 6.1%
   c. 5.3%
   d. 7.8%
   e. Psychiatric
3. 2.4%
4. a. 3.8%
   b. 2.8%
   c. 3.1%
   d. 3.96% or 4.0%
5. 0.84% or 0.8%
6. a. 5.0%
   b. 4.0%
   c. 3.5%

23. Postop Death Rate:

1. 1.07%
2. 2.66%

24. Anesthesia Death Rate:

1. a. 0.11%
   b. 0.65%
   c. 2.16%
   d. 1.68%
2. a. 0%
   b. 0.77%
   c. 3.44%
   d. 2.32%

25. Maternal Death Rate:

1. 0.24%
2. 0.15%
3. 0.31%

26. Fetal Death Rate:

1. a. 0.83%
   b. 0.42%
2. a. 1.49%
   b. 0.77%
3. a. 1.29%
   b. 0.32%

Chapter 5 Test

1. Fetal death
2. a. Less than 20 weeks
   b. From 20 to 28 weeks
   c. Twenty-eight weeks or more
3. a. Less than 500 grams
   b. From 501 through 1000 grams
   c. 1001 grams or more
4. a. Fetal deaths

b. Deaths under 48 hours and fetal deaths
c. Early fetal deaths
d. Deaths more than 10 days postoperative
5. Postoperative deaths—patients operated on
   Anesthetic deaths—anesthesia administered
   Fetal deaths—births plus intermediate and
   late fetal deaths
6. Net death rate
7. No
8. a. 4.83%
   b. 1.22%
9. 5.76%
10. 0.21%
11. 0.54%
12. 0.08%
13. 1.75%
14. a. 1.03%
    b. 2.60%
15. a. 7.86%
    b. 7.07%
    c. 1.25%
16. a. 2.67%
    b. 6.52%
17. a. 2.31%
    b. 0.90%
    c. 0.31%
18. a. 0.86%
    b. 0.32%
    c. 0.76%
    d. 2.19%
19. a. 3.51%
    b. 1.88%
    c. 1.87%
    d. 2.17%
    e. Obstetrics
    f. Surgery
    g. 4.35%
    h. 1.30%
    i. 0.87%
    j. 3.51%

CHAPTER 6

Self-Tests

27. Hospital Autopsy:

1. Yes	7. No
2. Yes	8. Yes
3. No	9. Yes
4. Yes	10. Yes
5. Yes	11. No
6. No	

28. Gross Autopsy Rate:

1. a. 44.44%
   b. 2.26%

2. a. 38.89%
    b. 2.02%
3. a. 51.35%
    b. 2.91%
    c. 1.34%
29. Net Autopsy Rate:
1. a. 57.89%
    b. 50%
2. a. 38.71%
    b. 0.90%
    c. 33.33%
    d. 1.29%
    e. 0.42%
    f. 0.52%
30. Hospital Autopsy Rate:
1. a. 66.67%
    b. 50%
    c. 1.46%
2. a. 66.67%
    b. 60%
    c. 1.84%
3. a. 64.71%
    b. 57.14%
    c. 57.14%
4. a. 75%
    b. 57.14%
    c. 66.67%
31. Newborn Autopsy Rate:
1. a. 50%
    b. 0.89%
2. 100%
3. 100%
32. Fetal Autopsy Rate:
1. a. 50%
    b. 100%
    c. 0.85%
    d. 0.41%
2. a. 50%
    b. 1.13%
    c. 0%
    d. 0.29%

Chapter 6 Test
1. Hospital autopsy rates
2. Hospital pathologist or designated physician on the hospital staff
3. Violent deaths—homicides, suicides, murder, drowning, and those suspected to be the result of foul play
4. Fetal deaths
5. Combined
6. No
7. Unautopsied coroner's cases
8. a. 12.82%

b. 13.51%
c. 17.95%
9. a. 50%
    b. 35.71%
    c. 37.50%
    d. 46.15%
    e. 89.31%
    f. 83.45%
10. a. 42.86%
    b. 46.15%
    c. 58.82%
    d. 66.67%
    e. 100%
11. a. 29.27%
    b. 33.33%
    c. 50%
    d. 28.57%
    e. 33.33%
    f. 50%
12. a. 0%
    b. 35.90%
    c. 38.89%
    d. 30.77%
    e. 40%

CHAPTER 7

Self-Tests
33. LOS:

1. 1 day	6. 37 days
2. 1 day	7. 15 days
3. 14 days	8. 75 days
4. 7 days	9. 118 days
5. 2 days	10. 522 days

34. Average LOS:
1. a. 7 days
    b. 3 days
    c. 6.20 days
2. a. 8.06 days
    b. 2.21 days
3. a. 10.6 days   c. 9.67 days
    b. 15 days   d. 2.5 days
4. a. A&C = 5.05 days
    b. 4.91 days
    c. 7.65 days
    d. 2.93 days
    e. 2.94 days
    f. 2.50 days
    g. 81.23%
    h. 45.54%
5. a. 5.01 days
    b. July–September
    c. January–March
6. a. 6.37 days

b. Neurosurgery

c. EENT

d.	EENT	2.17 days
	Neurosurgery	9.29 days
	Thoracic	8.09 days
	Abdominal	6.97 days
	GU	5.97 days
	Other	4.23 days

35. NB:

  1. a. 2.09 days

    b. 87.74%

  2. a. 2.62 days   d. 58%

    b. 2.69 days   e. 62%

    c. 2.5 days   f. 54%

  3. a. 2.6 days

    b. 2.5 days

    c. 2.67 days

    d. 7 lb 8 oz

    e. 8 lb 10 oz

    f. 6 lb 15 oz

Chapter 7 Test

1. Day of discharge
2. Yes—patient hospitalized over one year
3. Length of stay for all patients in a given period
4. a. Yes
   b. No
5. A physician writes an order allowing the patient to leave the hospital and to return at a specified time the patient is absent at the census-taking time.
6. a. Discharge days; average length of stay
   b. Inpatient service days; inpatient census; bed occupancy percentage
7. The patient is still hospitalized
8. a. 1 day   d. 18 days   g. 7 days
   b. 1 day   e. 11 days   h. 3 days
   c. 69 days   f. 202 days   i. 397 days
9. a. 5.35 days d. 50%
   b. 3.84 days e. 89.26%
   c. 0.82%   f. 75.33%
10. a. 3, 15, 11, 31, 3, 3, 6, 10, 6, 1, 1, 5, 4, 7, 5
    b. 7.71 days
    c. 3 days
    d. 8.33 days
    e. 7 days
    f. 5 days
11. a. A&C = 5.02 days; NB = 3.74 days

b.	Medical	4.88 days
	Surgical	7.59 days
	Obstetrics	3.93 days
	Gynecology	4.01 days
	Urology	4.21 days
	Newborn	3.74 days

c. Bed = 81.35%

   Bassinet = 75.05%

d. 2.51%

12. a. 5.23 days

   b. September

   c. June

   d. 83.84%

   e. February

   f. July

   g. 3.10%

CHAPTER 8

Self-Tests

36. C-Section/OB:

  1. 1.35%

  2. a. 59

    b. 56

    c. 0

    d. 30.36%

  3. a. 68

    b. 1

    c. 69

    d. 23.19%

  4. a. (Delivered for first time divided by total deliveries) × 100

    b. 23.33%

    c. (C-section for first delivery divided by number delivered for the first time) × 100

    d. 33.3%

    e. 14.29%

37. Consultation Rates:

  1. a. 48.05%

    b. 24.06%

  2. a. 27.05%

    b. Newborn

    c. Surgical

  3. a. 28.57%

    b. 21.43%

    c. 3.57%

    d. 100%

    e. 80.65%

38. Hospital Infection Rate:

  1. 0.35%

  2. a. 1.86%

    b. 3.53%

    c. Orthopedics

    d. Medical

39. Postoperative Infection Rate:

  1. a. 2.44%   d. 28.87%

    b. 1.45%   e. 86.91%

    c. 1.41%   f. 0.60%

  2. a. 1.20%   e. 0.59%

b. 1.62% f. 2.91%
c. 1.16% g. 1.76%
d. 27.91% h. 82.66%
3. a. March f. 90.22%
   b. 1.23% g. 0.86%
   c. 0.30% h. 32.48 = 32 patients
   d. 1.14% i. 2.01%
   e. March
4. a. 30
   b. 36.29 = 36 patients
   c. 90.71%
   d. 6.45%
   e. 2.70%
   f. 3.03%
   g. 2.78%

40. Turnover Rate:
1. a. 76.28% e. 88.51%
   b. 7.64 days f. 3.93 days
   c. 36.72 g. 83
   d. 36.44 h. 83.21

Chapter 8 Test

1. a. 0.98%
   b. 100%
   c. 30.34%
2. a. 21.96%
   b. Surgery
   c. 1.16%
   d. Surgery
   e. 1.96%
   f. 27.27%
3. a. 23.48%
   b. 2.13%
   c. CV
4. a. 230 d. 26.19%
   b. 252 e. 7.47%
   c. 2
5. a. 27.85% d. 2.46% g. 0.39%
   b. 0.60% e. 12% h. 0.30%
   c. 27.16% f. 0.46% i. 34.65%
6. a. 11 d. 25% g. 7 lb 3 oz
   b. 1 e. 8.33% h. 7 lb 2 oz
         f. 63.64%

UNIT I EXAM

1. a. Period A: A&C = 168.56 NB = 16.2
           B: A&C = 187.43 NB = 16.38
           C: A&C = 176.02 NB = 16.30
        Year: A&C = 177.41 NB = 16.29
   b. Period A: A&C = 84.28% NB = 54%
           B: A&C = 85.20% NB = 54.61%
           C: A&C = 83.82% NB = 54.32%
        Year: A&C = 84.45% NB = 54.31%

c. Gross: 2.43%
   Net: 1.60%
   NB: 0.46%
d. NB: 55.56%
   Gross: 40.28%
   Net: 42.77%
e. A&C: 5.05 days
   NB: 3.07 days
2. a. A&C: 176.2
      NB: 27.2
   b. A&C: 88.10%
      NB: 77.71%
   c. Gross: 2.11%
      Net: 1.36%
      NB: 1.66%
      Postoperative: 0.94%
      Anesthesia: 0.30%
      Maternal: 0.96%
      Fetal: 2.58%
   d. NB: 33.33%
      Fetal: 20%
      Gross: 32%
      Net: 36.36%
   e. 27.41%
   f. Hospital: 1.10%;
      Postoperative: 0.31%
   g. A&C = 5.32 days; NB = 3.92 days
3. a. Yes d. Yes
   b. Yes e. No
   c. No f. No
4. 100
5. Total number of deaths
6. Total number of deaths
7. ISPD (Inpatient service days)
8. Discharge days
9. a. (1) 62.77 patients
      (2) 38.28 patients
   b. (1) 19
      (2) 127.42
      (3) 22.40
   c. (1) 94.85%
      (2) 90.43%
      (3) 91.81%
   d. (1) 0.59% (4) 0.10% (7) 0.90%
      (2) 0.85% (5) 0.48%
      (3) 0.05% (6) 1.75%
   e. (1) 30.23% (3) 51.61% (5) 16.67%
      (2) 28.89% (4) 25%
   f. 19.86%
   g. (1) 78.51%
      (2) 13.56%
   h. (1) 5.76%
      (2) 2.55%

i. (1) 5.07 days
   (2) 3.34 days
   (3) 5.25 days
j. Period B
k. 80.95%
l. 66.67%

CHAPTER 9

Self-Tests

41. Frequency Distribution:
1. (1a) 3   (1b) 15
   (2a) 5   (2b) 13
   (3a) 15   (3b) 13
   (4a) 2   (4b) 13
2. a. 11   c. 12
   b. 39   d. 15
3. a. 227   b. 122   c. 0.63
4. a. 55.5–58.4
   b. 24.5%–75.4%
   c. 0.275–0.304
5. 8, 28; 6, 20; 7, 14; 7, 7
6. Lower interval limits, 85-89
   Upper interval limits, 165-169

Chapter 9 Test

1. a. 7
   b. 15
   c. low = 0–6; high = 98–104 (15 intervals)
      (0–6; 7–13; 14–20; 21–27; 28–34; 35–41;
      42–48; 49–55; 56–62; 63–69; 70–76; 77–83;
      84–90; 91–97; 98–104)
2. a. low = 0–4; high = 90–94
   b. 19 intervals
3. low = gain of 10 to 14 lbs; high = loss of 71
   to 75 lbs;
   frequencies: 2, 1, 2, 1, 2, 1, 5, 2, 5, 5, 4, 5, 3,
   l4, 0, 1, 1, 1
   cumulative frequency: 2, 3, 5, 6, 8, 9, 14, 16,
   21, 26, 30, 35, 38, 42, 42, 43, 44, 45
4. low = 10–14; high = 85–89
5. low = 50–74; high = 425–449
6. low = 0–2; high = 42–44; 15 intervals
7. a. 248
   b. 13
   c. low = 130–149; high = 370–389
   d. 2, 3, 12, 17, 18, 24, 10, 9, 4, 0, 0, 0, 1
      2, 5, 17, 34, 52, 76, 86, 95, 99, 99, 99, 99, 100
8. a. 33
   b. 17

c. low = 72–73; high = 104–105; 17 intervals
   tallies: 1, 3, 4, 3, 7, 7, 10, 6, 11, 9, 5, 5, 5, 3,
   3, 1, 1
   cumulative frequency: 1, 4, 8, 11, 18, 25,
   35, 41, 52, 61, 66, 71, 76, 79, 82, 83, 84

CHAPTER 10

Self-Tests

42. **Central Tendency:**
    Arithmetic Mean = 10.8 or 11
43. Weighted Mean = 87.14
44. Grouped Mean = 61 years of age
45. Median = 54.5
46. Mode: a. 73   b. 77   c. 77

Chapter 10 Test

1. a. 96   b. 93.67   c. 97
2. 89
3. Mean
4. Median
5. a. 86
   b. 14.5 days
   c. 9.5 days
   d. 2 days
   e. 14.83 days
   f. (1) 4 days   (4) 14 days
      (2) 21 days   (5) 3 days
      (3) 35 days
   g. (1) 87th percentile (76 out of 86)
      (2) 71st percentile (62 out of 86)
      (3) 53rd percentile (46 out of 86)
   h. 57%
   i. 28%
   j. 78th percentile
6. a. Left   b. Left
7. Left to right—mean, median, mode

CHAPTER 11

Self-Tests

47. **Graph:**

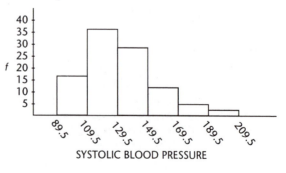

SYSTOLIC BLOOD PRESSURE

48. Graph

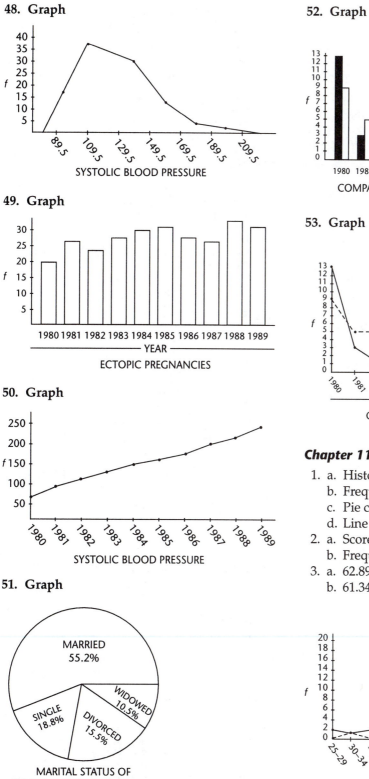

SYSTOLIC BLOOD PRESSURE

49. Graph

ECTOPIC PREGNANCIES

50. Graph

SYSTOLIC BLOOD PRESSURE

51. Graph

MARITAL STATUS OF
HOSPITALIZED PATIENTS OVER
AGE 14 IN THE PAST YEAR

MARRIED
55.2%

WIDOWED
10.5%

DIVORCED
15.5%

SINGLE
18.8%

52. Graph

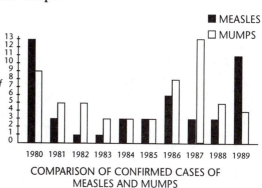

■ MEASLES
□ MUMPS

COMPARISON OF CONFIRMED CASES OF
MEASLES AND MUMPS

53. Graph

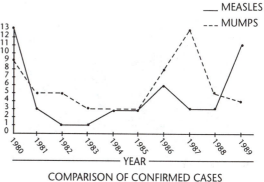

MEASLES
MUMPS

COMPARISON OF CONFIRMED CASES
OF MEASLES AND MUMPS

Chapter 11 Test

1. a. Histogram
   b. Frequency polygon
   c. Pie chart
   d. Line graph
2. a. Score limits
   b. Frequency
3. a. 62.89 years
   b. 61.34 years

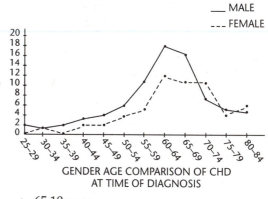

MALE
FEMALE

GENDER AGE COMPARISON OF CHD
AT TIME OF DIAGNOSIS

c. 65.10 years

4.

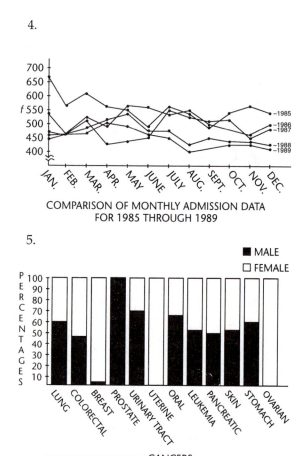

COMPARISON OF MONTHLY ADMISSION DATA
FOR 1985 THROUGH 1989

5.

■ MALE
□ FEMALE

GENDER COMPARISON OF
REPORTED CANCER PERCENTAGES

6.

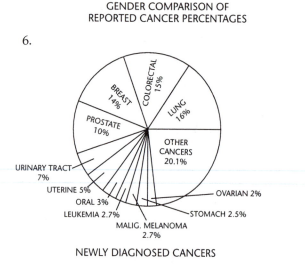

NEWLY DIAGNOSED CANCERS

7.

DACRYOCYSTORHINOSTOMY	⚤
EPISTAXIS CONTROL	⚤⚤
ETHMOIDECTOMY	⚤⚤
LARYNGECTOMY (RADICAL)	⚤⚤
LARYNGOSCOPY/ TRACHEOSCOPY	⚤⚤⚤
MASTOIDECTOMY	⚤⚤⚤
MYRINGOPLASTY	⚤⚤
MYRINGOTOMY WITH INSERTION OF TUBE	⚤⚤⚤
PHARYNGOPLASTY	⚤
RHINOPLASTY	⚤
SEPTOPLASTY	⚤⚤⚤⚤
SIALADENECTOMY	⚤⚤⚤⚤
STAPEDECTOMY	⚤
THYROIDECTOMY	⚤
TONSILLECTOMY WITH ADENOIDECTOMY (T&A)	⚤⚤⚤⚤⚤⚤⚤⚤⚤⚤⚤⚤⚤⚤⚤⚤⚤⚤⚤⚤⚤⚤⚤⚤⚤⚤⚤⚤⚤
TONSILLECTOMY WITHOUT ADENOIDECTOMY	⚤⚤⚤⚤⚤⚤⚤⚤

UNIT II EXAM

1. a. (1) 55.14 years
      (2) 54 years
      (3) 56.22 years
      (4) 59.53 years
      (5) 56.76 years

   b. 59 years

   c. 59 years

   d.

Score Limits	Mid pt.	Male Freq.	Male *cf.*	Female Freq.	Female *cf.*	Combined freq.	*cf.*
100+	105		17		18	0	35
90–99	95		17		18	0	35
80–89	85	// = 2	17	/// = 3	18	5	35
70–79	75	// = 2	15	/ = 1	15	3	30
60–69	65	// = 2	13	//// = 4	14	6	27
50–59	55	//// = 4	11	~~////~~ = 5	10	9	21
40–49	45	//// = 4	7	// = 2	5	6	12
30–39	35	// = 2	3	/ = 1	3	3	6
20–29	25		1	/ = 1	2	1	3
10–19	15		1		1	0	2
0–9	5	/ = 1	1	/ = 1	1	2	2

   e. 10

   f. 55.76 years

   g.

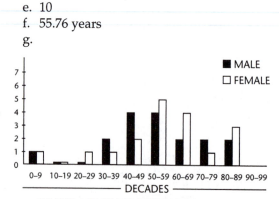

■ MALE
□ FEMALE

GENDER AGE COMPARISON AT TIME OF DEATH

2.

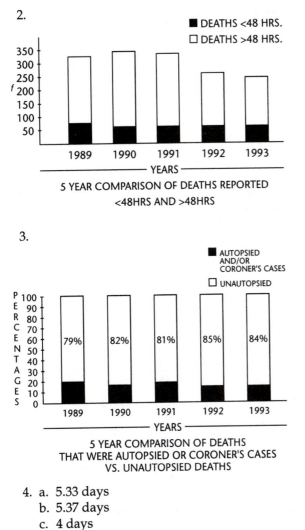

5 YEAR COMPARISON OF DEATHS REPORTED
<48HRS AND >48HRS

3.

5 YEAR COMPARISON OF DEATHS
THAT WERE AUTOPSIED OR CORONER'S CASES
VS. UNAUTOPSIED DEATHS

4. a. 5.33 days
    b. 5.37 days
    c. 4 days
    d. Both 2 and 3 with a frequency of 13 each
    e. (1) 95th percentile
       (2) 87th percentile
    f. 1 to 33 = 32 scores
    g.

LOS	f	cf	Mid pt.	f × Mid pt.	
33–34	1	75	33.5	33.5	a. $\frac{400}{75}$ = 5.33 days
31–32	0	74			
29–30	0	74			b. $\frac{402.5}{75}$ = 5.37 days
27–28	0	74			
25–26	0	74			
23–24	0	74			
21–22	1	74	21.5	21.5	
19–20	1	73	19.5	19.5	
17–18	0	72			
15–16	1	72	15.5	15.5	
13–14	4	71	13.5	54.0	
11–12	1	67	11.5	11.5	
9–10	1	66	9.5	9.5	
7–8	6	65	7.5	45.0	
5–6	14	59	5.5	77.0	
3–4	24	45	3.5	84.0	
1–2	21	21	1.5	31.5	
	75			402.5	

5. a. 3.1 years
    b. 1 year
    c. Both 1 day and 1 year—frequency of 8
    d. 5.24 years
    e. 6.52 days
    f. 4 days
    g. 1 day
    h. 1 year

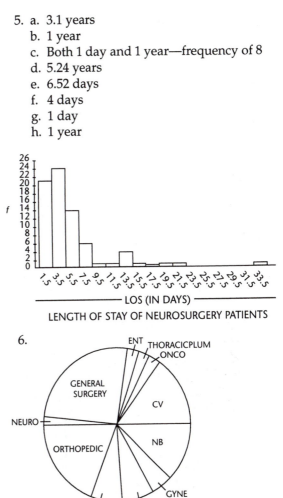

LENGTH OF STAY OF NEUROSURGERY PATIENTS

6.

PERCENTAGE OF SURGICAL
PROCEDURES DURING
THE PAST SIX MONTHS

REFERENCES

1. American Medical Record Association, *Glossary of Health Care Terms*, (Chicago: AMRA, 1986).

2. Huffman, Edna K., RRA, *Medical Record Management*, 9th edition, revised by AMRA (Rita Finnegan and Margaret Amatayakul), (Berwyn, IL: Physicians Record Company, 1990).

Index

A&C. *See* Adults and children
A&D. *See* Admitted and discharged
Abbreviations, 7–8
  clinical units, 7–8
  non-official, 8
  patient care, 7
  statistical, 7
Aborted fetus, 70, 194
Abortion, 68
Actual class limits, 140
Admission data, 58, 96
Admitted after delivery, 194
Admitted and discharged (A&D), 26
Adults and children (A&C), 30
  average daily inpatient census, 33–34
  occupancy percentage, 43–44
Against medical advice (AMA), 58
Ambulatory care patients, 23
Anesthesia death, 65, 66, 193
Antepartum, 68
Arithmetic mean, 150
Autopsy, 80, 193
Autopsy rates, 79–91
  fetal, 90
  general information, 81–82
  gross, 83
  hospital, 86–87
  net, 85
  newborn, 89
  terms, 80–81
Average, 14
Average census, 32–34
  A&C, 33–34
  average daily inpatient census (average daily census), 32–33, 192
  clinical unit, 34
  NB, 34
Average length of stay, 96, 99
  adults and children, 100
  newborn, 103
Averaging, 14–15

Bar graph/bar chart, 172–180
  as comparison graph, 178–180
  construction of, 173–174
Bassinet statistics, 30
Bassinet turnover rate, 121
Bed/bassinet count day terms, 42–43
Bed complement, 41
Bed occupancy day, 27
Beds
  disaster, 42, 44
  excluded, 42
  statistics, 30
  unit vs. totals, 42
Bed turnover rate, 120–121
  bassinet turnover rate, 121
  direct bed turnover rate, 121
  indirect bed turnover rate, 121
  usefulness of turnover rates, 121
Bell-shaped curve, 150, 153
Bilaterally symmetrical curves, 153–154
  bell-shaped curve, 150, 153
  flat curves, 153, 154
  peaked curves, 153, 154
Bimodal curve, 157
Bimodal distribution, 152

Census, 22–36, 192
  average, 32–34
  calculation tips, 29–30
  collection and terms, 23–30
  defined, 23
  inpatient, 23, 26
  taking, 24–26
Census day, 27
Census taking, 24–26
  central collection, 25
  reporting, 25
  time of day, 24
  transfers, 25–26
Census-taking time (CTT), 24, 25, 26,27, 28, 105
Centiles, 158

Cesarean section rate, 111–112
Change in bed count during a period, 48
Chart, 164
Class, as related to frequency distribution
  boundaries, 140
  interval, 139, 140, 141
  length, 140
  limits, 140
  size, 140–141
  width, 140
Class intervals, in histogram, 168
Clinical units, 24
  average daily census, 34
  occupancy percentage for a period, 46
Comparison graphs, 177–181
  bar graphs, 178–180
  line graphs, 180–181
Comparison of percentage bar graph, 179
Component part graph, 178
Computerized data
  accuracy, 5
  use, 5
Computing with a percentage, 18–19
Constant, 4
Consultation rate, 113–114
Continuous data, 166
Continuous quality improvement (CQI), 8
Continuous variable, 4, 140
Conversion to another form, 17–18
  decimal to percentage, 17
  fraction to percentage, 17
  percentage to decimal, 17
  percentage to fraction, 17
  ratio to percentage, 17
Coroner's case, 80–81
Counts, 6
CTT. *See* Census-taking time

Cumulative frequency, 141–142, 159–160
  converted into percentile, 159–160
  related to percentiles, 159
  steps in cumulating, 141–142
Curves of frequency distributions,
    153–157
  bilaterally symmetrical curves,
    153–154
  skewed curves, 154–156
  other curves, 156–157

Daily inpatient bed occupancy
    percentage, 43
Daily inpatient census (DIPC), 26, 27,
    28, 192
  recording, 28
Daily newborn bassinet occupancy
    percentage, 44
Data, 12
  computerized, 5
  continuous, 4, 166
  defined, 2
  discrete, 4
  graphing, 163–181
  grouped, 4–5, 137, 151
  patient, 5–6
  ungrouped, 4
  uses of, 8
Data base (data bank), 2, 12
Data processing, 2
Dated, 6
Day on leave of absence, 105, 192
DD. *See* Discharge days
Dead on arrival (DOA), 29, 59
Death, 28–29
  anesthesia, 65, 66, 193
  DOA (dead on arrival), 29, 59
  fetal, 29, 59–60
  inpatient, 58–59
  maternal, 67, 68, 193
  non-patient, 59–60
  outpatient, 29, 58, 59
  postoperative, 65, 193
Deciles, 158
Decimal, 13
Delivered in the hospital, 194
Delivery, 68, 111, 194
Denominator, 12
Descriptive statistics, 5
Diagnoses, 6
Diagram, 164
DIPC (daily inpatient census), 26, 27
Direct bed turnover rate, 121
Direct maternal death, 67, 193
Disaster beds, 42
  and occupancy rates, 44
Discharge data, 58, 61, 62, 96
Discharge days (DD), 96, 98
  importance of, 98
  totaling, 98
Discharges, 28
  deaths, 28
  live, 28, 58
Discrete data, 4
DOA (dead on arrival), 29, 59

Early fetal death, 59, 193
Emergency room (ER) death, 59
Excluded beds, 42

Fetal autopsy rate, 90
Fetal death, 29, 59–60, 193
Fetal death rate, 70–72
  deaths included in rate, 70
Flat curves, 153, 154
Formulae, 196–199
  autopsy rates, 198–199
  census, 196
  death rates, 197–198
  length of stay, 199
  occupancy, 197
  other rates, 199
  rate formula, 197
Fraction, 12–13
  denominator, 12
  numerator, 12
  quotient, 13
Frequency, 141
Frequency distribution, 136–146
  arranged scores, 138
  creating, 142–145
  curves of , 153–157
  grouped, 137–138
  terms related to, 138–142
  ungrouped, 137
Frequency distribution, plotting,
    164–165
  axes, 165
  scale proportion, 165
  vertical scale, 165
Frequency polygon, 170
  advantage of, 170
  compared with histogram, 171
  construction of, 170, 171
  superimposing two frequency of
    polygons, 171–172
  when to use, 170

Glossary of Health Care Terms, 23, 24
Graph, 164
Graphing data, 163–181
  bar graph/bar chart, 172–174, 178–180
  comparison graph, 177, 181
  frequency polygon, 170, 171
  histogram, 165–169, 171
  line graph, 174–175, 180–181
  pictograph/pictogram, 176–177
  pie graph/pie chart, 175–176
  plotting a frequency distribution,
    164–165
Gross autopsy rate, 83
Gross death rate, 60–61
Grouped data, 4, 137, 151
  computing mean from, 151
Grouped frequency distribution, 137
  purpose of, 138

Health Information Department, 3
Histogram, 165–169
  compared with frequency polygon,
    171
  construction of, 166–169, 171
Home care patients, 23
  autopsy, 80
Horizontal axis, 164, 165
Hospital
  departments, 24
  patients, 23–24
  services, 24
  units, 24

Hospital autopsy, 80, 81–82, 194
  consent, 82
  data on adults/children and
    newborns combined, 82
  Excluded deaths, 81
  legal cases, 82
  report requirements, 81
  where performed, 81
  who is included, 81
  who performs, 81
Hospital autopsy rate (adjusted), 86–87
Hospital fetal death, 59–60, 193
  designated by gestational age, 59
  designated by gram weight, 59
Hospital infection rate, 115–116
Hospital inpatient autopsy, 80, 194
Hospital live birth, 195
Hospital patients, 23–24, 191
  ambulatory care patients, 23
  boarder, 191
  inpatients, 23, 191
  newborn inpatient, 191
  outpatients, 23–24, 191

Indirect bed turnover rate, 121
Indirect maternal death, 67–68, 193
Induced termination of pregnancy, 194
Infant death, 193
Infant death rate, 62
Infant mortality rate, 62
Infection rates, 115–120
  hospital infection rate (nosocomial
    rate), 115–116
  postoperative infection rate, 116–117
Inferential statistics, 5
Inpatient (IP), 23
  adults and children (A&C), 30
  newborn (NB), 30
Inpatient admission, 192
Inpatient bassinet count day, 43, 192
Inpatient bed count, 41, 192
Inpatient bed count day, 43
Inpatient bed count days (total), 43, 193
Inpatient bed occupancy percentage for
    a period, 45
Inpatient bed occupancy ratio, 43, 193
Inpatient census, 23, 192
Inpatient day, 27
Inpatient discharge, 192
Inpatient hospitalization, 191
Inpatient service day (IPSD), 26–28,
    192
  recording, 28
  total, 28, 192
Institutional death rate, 61
Interhospital transfer, 25
Intermediate fetal death, 59, 193
Intrahospital transfer, 25
IPSD. *See* Inpatient service day

J-shaped curve, 157

Late fetal death, 59, 193
Leave of absence day, 105, 192
Length of stay (LOS)
  average, 96, 99
  calculating, 96–97
  defined, 96, 194
Line graph, 174–175
  as comparison graph, 180–181

Live discharges, 28
Local area network (LAN), 5
LOS. *See* Length of stay
Lower class limit, 140

Maternal death, 67–68, 193
  direct, 67
  included in hospital statistics, 68
  indirect, 67–68
  not included in hospital statistics, 68
Maternal death rates, 67–70
Mean, 150–152
  arithmetic, 150
  computed from grouped data, 151
  weighted, 150–151
Measures of central tendency, 149–160
  and effects of skewness, 155
  mean, 150–152
  median, 152
  mode, 152
Medical care unit, 195
Medical consultation, 195
Medical examiner's case, 80–81
Medical Record Management (Huffman), 66
Medical services, 195
Medical staff unit, 195
Morbidity, 58
Morbidity rates. *See* Infection rates
Morgue, 81
Mortality, 58
Mortality (death) rates, 57–73
  fetal (stillborn), 70–72
  gross, 60–61
  helpful hints for calculating, 62
  maternal, 67–70
  net (or institutional), 61
  newborn, 62
  surgical, 65–67
  terms, 58–60
Multimodal curve, 157

NB. *See* Newborn
Neonatal death, 193
Neonatal periods, 195
Net autopsy rate, 85
Net death rate, 61
Newborn (NB), 30
  autopsy rate, 89
  average daily inpatient census, 34
  bassinet count, 41, 192
  death rate, 62
  occupancy percentage, 44
  occupancy percentage for a period, 46
Normal bell-shaped curve, 150, 153
Nosocomial infection, 115
Nosocomial rate, 115–116
Not delivered (pregnant woman), 111, 195
Numerator, 12
Nursing homes (extended care facilities), 23

Obstetrics, 194
Occupancy, percentage of, 40–51
  bed/bassinet count day terms, 42–43
  bed/bassinet count terms, 41
  beds, categories of, 42
  change in bed count during a period, 48–50

  for a period, 45–48
  rate formula, 41–42
  ratio/percentage, 43–45
Occupancy ratio/percentage
  adults and children, 43–44
  all beds occupied, 43–44
  and disaster beds, 44
  newborn, 44
  normal, 44
Outpatient (OP), 23–24
  autopsy, 80
  death, 29

Partum, 68
Pathologist, 81
Patient data, types of, 5–6
  counts, 6
  dates, 6
  diagnoses, 6
  procedures, 6
  test results, 6
  treatment outcomes and assessments, 6
Patient day, 27
Peaked curves, 153, 154
Pediatric patient, 191
Percentage, 13, 158–160
  computing with, 18–19
Percentage component part graph, 178
Percentile, 158
  conversion of cumulative frequency into, 159–160
  importance of, 158–159
  related to cumulative frequency, 159
  weakness of, 59
Percentile rank, 158
Percentile score, 158
Perinatal death, 193
Period, 27
Pictograph/pictogram, 176–177
Pie graph/pie chart, 175–176
Population, 3
Postoperative death, 65, 193
Postoperative death rate, 65
Postoperative infection rate, 116–117
Postpartum, 68
Pregnancy termination, 194
Premature birth, 60, 195
Procedures, 6
Proportion, 14
Puerperium, 68, 194

Qualitative variables, 4
Quality assessment, 8
Quantitative data, 166
Quantitative variable, 4
Quartiles, 158
Quotient, 13

Range, 139
Rank, 158
Rate, 13–14
Rate formula, 41–42
Ratio, 14
Raw score limits, 140
Real class limits, 140
Reverse J-shaped curve, 157
Rounding data, 15–16

Sample, 2–4
Scale proportion, 165
Score limits, 140
Side-by-side comparison graphs, 178
Skewed curves, 154–156
  effect of skewness on measure of central tendency, 155
  reporting averages, 156
  reporting measures of central tendency from a skewed distribution, 155
  skewed to left (negative skewness), 154
  skewed to right (positive skewness), 154
Special care unit, 195
Statistical data, reporting, 1–9
  terms and definitions, 3–5
Statistics
  defined, 2
  descriptive, 5
  inferential, 5
Stillborn infant, 29, 193
Stillborn rate, 70
Surgical death rates, 65–67
  anesthesia, 66
  postoperative, 65
Surgical operation, 117, 195
Surgical procedure, 116–117, 195
Symmetrical curves, 153–154

Test results, 6
Tissue specimens, 81
Total inpatient service days, 28, 192
  recording, 28
Total length of stay, 96, 98, 194
Total quality management (TQM), 8
Totals, 27
Transferred-in (TRF-in), 25, 28
Transferred-out (TRF-out), 25, 28
Transfers, 25–26
  counting, 26
  interhospital, 25, 192
  intrahospital, 25, 192
Treatment outcomes and assessments, 6
True class units, 140

Unautopsied coroner's cases, 81
Undelivered (pregnant woman), 68
Ungrouped data, 4
Ungrouped frequency distribution, 137
Unimodal distribution, 152
Unit of measure, 27
Units
  clinical, 24
  hospital, 24
Upper class limit, 140
U-shaped curve, 157

Variable, 4
  continuous, 4
  qualitative, 4
  quantitative, 4
Vertical axis, 164, 165
Vertical scale, 165

Weighted mean, 150–151